T0349470

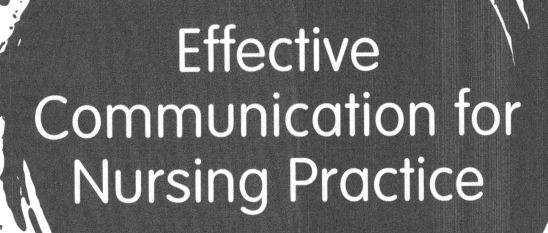

Effective Communication for Nursing Practice

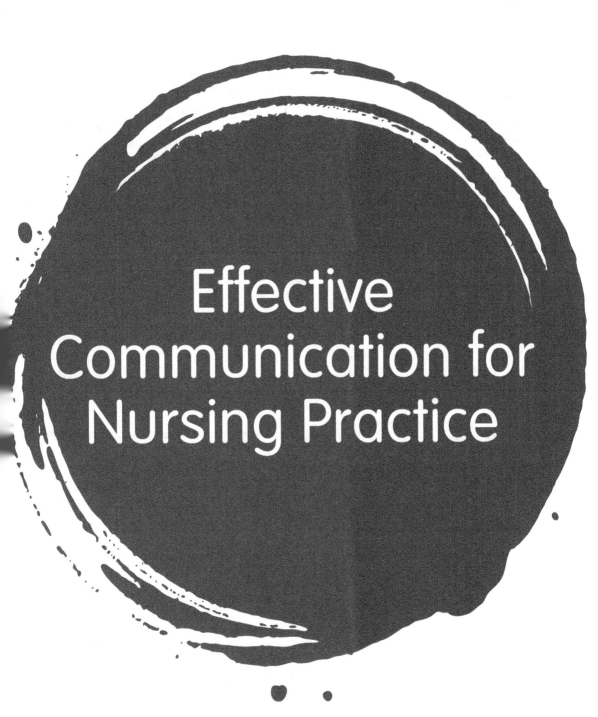

Effective Communication for Nursing Practice

Naomi Anna Watson

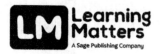

Learning Matters
A Sage Publishing Company
1 Oliver's Yard
55 City Road
London EC1Y 1SP

Sage Publications Inc.
2455 Teller Road
Thousand Oaks, California 91320

Sage Publications India Pvt Ltd
B 1/I 1 Mohan Cooperative Industrial Area
Mathura Road
New Delhi 110 044

Sage Publications Asia-Pacific Pte Ltd
3 Church Street
#10-04 Samsung Hub
Singapore 049483

Editor: Martha Cunneen
Development editor: Ruth Lilly
Senior project editor: Chris Marke
Project management: Westchester Publishing
Services UK
Marketing manager: Ruslana Khatagova
Cover design: Sheila Tong
Typeset by: C&M Digitals (P) Ltd, Chennai, India
Printed in the UK

Library of Congress Control Number: 2024933077

British Library Cataloguing in Publication Data

A catalogue record for this book is available from the British Library

ISBN 978-1-5296-1189-2
ISBN 978-1-5296-1188-5 (pbk)

Contents

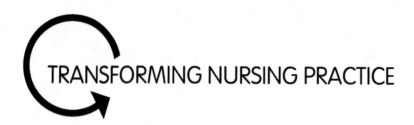

TRANSFORMING NURSING PRACTICE

Transforming Nursing Practice is a series tailor made for pre-registration student nurses. Each book in the series is:

 Affordable

 Mapped to the NMC Standards of proficiency for registered nurses

 Full of active learning features

 Focused on applying theory to practice

Each book addresses a core topic and they have been carefully developed to be simple to use, quick to read and written in clear language.

An invaluable series of books that explicitly relates to the NMC standards. Each book covers a different topic that students need to explore in order to develop into a qualified nurse... I would recommend this series to all Pre-Registered nursing students whatever their field or year of study.

LINDA ROBSON,
Senior Lecturer at Edge Hill University

Many titles in the series are on our recommended reading list and for good reason - the content is up to date and easy to read. These are the books that actually get used beyond training and into your nursing career.

EMMA LYDON,
Adult Student Nursing

ABOUT THE SERIES EDITORS

DR MOOI STANDING is an Independent Nursing Consultant (UK and International) and is responsible for the core knowledge, adult nursing and personal and professional learning skills titles. She is an experienced NMC Quality Assurance Reviewer of educational programmes and a Professional Regulator Panellist on the NMC Practice Committee. Mooi is also Board member of Special Olympics Malaysia, enabling people with intellectual disabilities to participate in sports and athletics nationally and internationally.

DR SANDRA WALKER is a Clinical Academic in Mental Health working between Southern Health Trust and the University of Southampton and responsible for the mental health nursing titles. She is a Qualified Mental Health Nurse with a wide range of clinical experience spanning more than 25 years.

BESTSELLING TEXTBOOKS

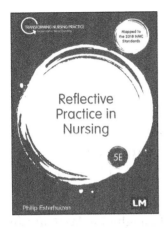

Reflective Practice in Nursing
5E
Philip Esterhuizen

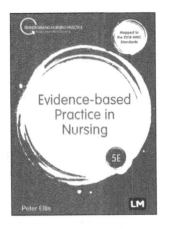

Evidence-based Practice in Nursing
5E
Peter Ellis

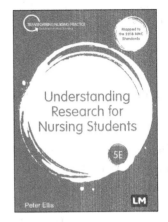

Understanding Research for Nursing Students
5E
Peter Ellis

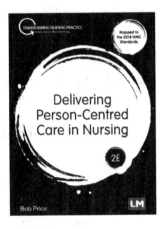

Delivering Person-Centred Care in Nursing
2E
Bob Price

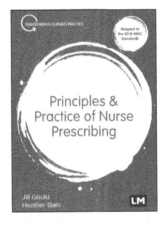

Principles & Practice of Nurse Prescribing
Jill Gould
Heather Bain

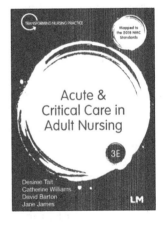

Acute & Critical Care in Adult Nursing
3E
Desiree Tait
Catherine Williams
David Barton
Jane James

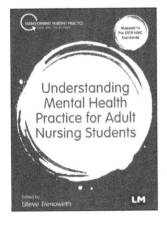

Understanding Mental Health Practice for Adult Nursing Students
Edited by
Steve Trenoweth

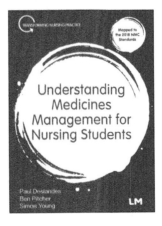

Understanding Medicines Management for Nursing Students
Paul Deslandes
Ben Pitcher
Simon Young

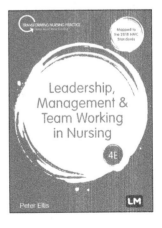

Leadership, Management & Team Working in Nursing
4E
Peter Ellis

You can find a full list of textbooks in the *Transforming Nursing Practice* series at
https://uk.sagepub.com/TNP-series

Acknowledgements

This book is dedicated to:

The memory of my maternal grandparents, the late Kathleen Beatrice and Levi Clarke who were never sparing in their 'can do, will do' supportive approach to life, living and doing one's best, no matter the test. They are always remembered with much love and affection.

Daughter Abeni and son-in-law Dwight Dinnall, son Joe and daughter-in-law Gifty and new baby Levi, named after great-grandpa, Levi Clarke, as a gentle reminder of our ancestor's 'can do, will do' approach to living.

Lorna Sterling who always quietly supported me by checking up on how the writing was going. Always a helpful reminder to keep going despite workload and other life distractions. It never failed to get me back on track. Thank you.

My colleagues who contributed to the book, thank you for delivering your chapters in good time.

Finally, last but by no means least, thank you to the Creator and Life Giver, for keeping me going despite the continuous distractions throughout this project of a number of family bereavements, including the loss of my dear mum, Minteena. Gone but never forgotten.

About the authors

Dr Naomi Anna Watson is Senior Lecturer in nursing at the Open University (OU). In her recent role as Deputy Associate Dean, teaching excellence, she contributed to the strategic direction of tutor development and student learning and teaching. She actively ensures quality outcomes that promote and improve student participation and success while also enabling a better understanding of the student voice. Her research interests span a range of areas across nursing education and practice, including the student experience at distance, health and social care debates about cultural competence, communication and professional practice, participation of African Caribbean people in nursing careers and Black women's health and wellbeing in the context of equity, diversity and inclusion (EDI). Her most recent research focuses on distance nursing education and the Covid-19 impact on professional practitioners of nursing and social work. Naomi is a doctoral supervisor, mentor and published author on primary care nursing, service user involvement, participation of African Caribbean students in nursing education, cultural competence and communication and diversity. She is also a keen lifelong volunteer, having supported several national, local and community charities, including Barnardo's, Diabetes UK, local secondary schools and The Girls' Network (TGN) as a mentor to disadvantaged girls.

Paulette Johnson is academic lead for access, participation and success at The Open University, in the WELS faculty. With a professional background in social work, her practice background has been in leadership and management across adult social care and criminal justice services, which has been the focus of her career over the last 20 years. Although now employed in a senior academic role, Paulette continues to support vulnerable adults in her capacity as Chair of a local charity. In her academic role, Paulette has undertaken several leadership roles at the OU as well as being a post graduate researcher and a doctoral candidate in the faculty. Her research and work interests include equality, diversity and inclusion, substance misuse, homelessness and co-production.

Dr Liz King qualified as a registered paediatric nurse in 2000 and has since gained copious experience in caring for children, young people and their families. Liz has been involved with pre-registration nurse education throughout her career in both clinical settings and in higher education as a nurse academic. Liz is currently a lecturer in children and young people's nursing at The Open University and holds a doctorate in education.

Dr Kay Norman is an experienced nursing academic and researcher who has published and presented on many aspects of communication. Kay's recent roles have included both strategic, management and clinical practice areas of responsibility. In her current role as head of teaching excellence for the School of Nursing and Midwifery at the University of Worcester, Kay leads and supports initiatives to continually improve student teaching and learning experiences. Her recent research has related to supporting international nursing students in clinical practice. She continues to supervise both undergraduate, postgraduate and doctoral students in their research studies. Kay is passionate about helping students to improve their communication skills and foster a curiosity in clinical practice to ultimately ensure patient safety.

Introduction

About this book

This book is an introductory text that aims to support you as an undergraduate student nurse or healthcare worker in developing and consolidating effective communication skills that are evidence based, relevant and important in current everyday nursing practice.

It aims to ensure that as a student nurse and healthcare professional, you are suitably prepared to deal with situations in clinical practice that require complex communication responses. It will contribute to measurable improvements in the quality of your therapeutic relationship with patients, their carers, other service users and other healthcare colleagues.

Why 'effective communication for nursing practice'?

The Code (NMC (Nursing and Midwifery Council), 2018) identifies communication as a very important underpinning skill that is required for appropriate care delivery practice. This is further embedded in the professional standards, which expect nurses, midwives and nursing associates to learn about communication as part of their standard curriculum and be able to apply their learning to clinical practice.

The text also responds directly to ongoing discontent with healthcare service delivery in a variety of settings, which have resulted in a number of public enquiries that identify problematic communication with patients, their carers and families as a major failure of the quality of services (see the Francis Report, (Francis, 2013)).

'The way you communicate', is the main theme of this book. It is intended to keep you alert and aware of the impact and implications of your personal communication style and of your responsibility to continuously improve and develop this essential skill throughout your learning and career as a qualified nurse and healthcare professional.

Pedagogical approach to the text

The book discusses and emphasises basic principles for effective communication that are sometimes overlooked in everyday practice, with the potential of causing harm to patients, their carers and families (see Grainger, 2013, Francis, 2013). The focus is on providing you with opportunities to practise the skills required to develop your competency in the clinical environment. In particular it will enable you to engage reflectively with all members of the multidisciplinary team, and support and encourage you to find and embed your own voice in the process. It outlines definitions and ensures that there are theoretical underpinnings to support knowledge, understanding and application to practice.

The book explores aspects of personal communication in relation to interpersonal perspectives, peer-to-peer communication and emotional intelligence. Using student activities and personal application, it will provide opportunities to develop self-awareness and reflective behaviours that will inform individual actions in practice and strengthen your levels of confidence in your own voice during everyday interactions. It will enable the development of your professional maturity by encouraging creative approaches to solving problems. It covers aspects of speaking with confidence as part of a professional discussion, with your supervisor and with your ward team as required for degree apprenticeship end-point assessment. It discusses the management of diverse encounters in clinical environments, for example with issues relating to some protected characteristics of the Equality Act (Legislation.gov.uk, 2010).

It explores communication across the lifespan emphasising children and young people, adults during the lifespan, midlife changes and the complexities of communication during likely midlife crises such as the menopause. It considers older people including those who live with dementia/Alzheimer's, vulnerable people including those who live with a learning disability or a mental disorder. It includes examples from a four-nations perspective to ensure that different approaches that speak to practice in each UK nation are recognised and acknowledged. It covers nursing and health perspectives of talking as therapy and ways of supporting the mental health and wellbeing of yourself, your peers, patients, families, carers and your professional colleagues.

The book includes interactive activities such as case studies and scenarios, with emphasis on patients, carers and service-user perspectives and their experiences of therapeutic communication while accessing healthcare and services for themselves and their families. It provides opportunities and encouragement for you to share your learning with your peers. It discusses possible scenarios and likely solutions to challenging issues both in acute hospital settings, emergency and out-of-hours urgent care environments, homecare and primary care practice. It explores communication and the digital world of technology from a global perspective. It discusses the issues that relate to 'race' and communication, focusing on inter-ethnic perspectives, cultural competence, cultural safety and cultural intelligence when dealing with diverse individuals and groups, as previously mentioned to link into the protected UK characteristics and human rights. It provides examples of potential barriers to successful communication and encourages compassionate communication. The aim is to situate this as an integral part of quality care delivery practice by suggesting ways of developing and managing these skills to enable and foster good professional practice.

Book structure

Chapter 1 introduces communication principles, their theoretical perspectives and overall contextual application in the global context. It covers concepts relating to initial healthcare requirements for students, such as peer-to-peer communication and its likely benefits for development and preparation for practice. It outlines varied definitions of communication and considers the theoretical perspectives, including the exploration of concepts such as the JOHARI window, emotional intelligence and self-awareness to individual understandings and application. It explores the impact of digital technologies and social media on your communication patterns.

Chapter 2 explores power relationships and their impact on effective communication including likely barriers to successful communication. It discusses communication and its potential to be applied as a form of social control and domination in the context of compliance, non-compliance/concordance and the social construction of health and illness. It outlines communication levels that are of relevance including therapeutic, interprofessional, political and administrative approaches, for example, whistleblowing. It provides insights to enable you to understand the importance of finding your voice and speaking with confidence in all healthcare environments.

Chapter 3 considers communication in different settings, for example, perspectives in primary and secondary care and community nursing settings, and home care. This also includes experiences in accident and emergency settings and urgent care facilities in the community. Student activities aim to enable application in clinical community environments.

Chapter 4 discusses inter-ethnic communication within the context of 'race' and cultural competence. The aim is to enable you to have a better understanding of the factors that influence interactions, in the context of global issues relating, for example, to the Black Lives Matter (BLM) movement and its application to aspects of social justice, health inequalities and antiracist practice. It provides opportunities for the exploration of ways to address current issues in nursing and health that will contribute to improving patient satisfaction and the quality of care that you deliver.

Chapter 5 outlines likely factors that influence communication within the multi-disciplinary team (MDT) and the wider healthcare team. Additionally, it considers communication skills that may be applied to foster opportunities for networking, leadership, management and innovation, including innovations in clinical practice.

Chapter 6 addresses communication as it applies to the needs and expectations of children, young people (CYP) their carers and families. It considers appropriate therapeutic approaches when working within this context using case studies and role play applications. Examples for exploration include safeguarding principles, children in care and the voice of the child.

Chapter 7 explores communication with adults with specific emphasis on life events including communication during pregnancy, birthing experiences, body image and body changes. Midlife issues such as divorce, loss, empty nest syndrome and the male/female menopause and overall menopausal impact on individuals are discussed.

Chapter 8 discusses communication with older people. It outlines communication principles as they apply to older people, including those who live with dementia and Alzheimer's disease. It explores the changes that occur in the experiences of older people, policy perspectives on care delivery and practice, adult safeguarding principles and effective communication strategies that can contribute to improving the quality of care and enabling independence for those who live with dementia and Alzheimer's.

Chapter 9 looks at the benefits of effective communication as it applies to supporting the mental health and wellbeing of patients, peers, staff and colleagues. It discusses the use and application of talking therapies and ways that these may be used to enable and improve mental health and wellbeing. Additionally, it provides an opportunity for you to examine your own self-care strategies, wellbeing and resilience.

Chapter 10 explores communication practice and experiences for people living with learning disability and considers strategies for effective and interactive interventions that promote positive behaviour outcomes and living and thriving independently.

Chapter 11 discusses communication and its application in relation to death, dying and bereavement. It interrogates issues relating to working with and supporting patients who are approaching the end of life and their carers and families.

Chapter 12 draws the book to a conclusion by pulling together a summary from the areas covered. It relates these to the overall theme of communication with compassion and the 6Cs. It provides a summary discourse to communication in clinical practice that will strengthen skills development and improve your professional practice.

Requirements for the NMC Standards of Proficiency for Registered Nurses

The Nursing and Midwifery Council (NMC) has established standards of proficiency to be met by applicants to different parts of the register, and these are the standards it considers necessary for safe and effective practice. This book is structured so that it will help you to understand and meet the proficiencies required for entry to the NMC register. The relevant proficiencies are presented at the start of each chapter so that you can clearly see which ones the chapter addresses. The proficiencies have been designed to be generic so apply to all fields of nursing and all care settings. This is because all nurses must be able to meet the needs of any person they encounter in their practice regardless of their stage of life or health challenges, whether these are mental, physical, cognitive, or behavioural.

This book includes the latest standards for 2018 onwards, taken from the *Future Nurse: Standards of Proficiency for Registered Nurses* (NMC, 2018).

Learning features

Learning from reading text is not always easy. Therefore, to provide variety and to assist with the development of independent learning skills and the application of theory to practice, this book contains activities such as case studies, scenarios, further reading, useful websites, including from a four-nations perspective, to enable you to apply your learning to the different nations of the UK and other materials to enable you to participate in your own learning. You will need to develop your own study skills and 'learn how to learn' to get the best from the material. This is an introductory book; it cannot provide all the answers – but instead provides a framework for your learning.

The activities in the book will help you to make sense of, and learn about, the material being presented. Some activities ask you to reflect on aspects of practice, your experience of it, or the people or situations you encounter. Reflection is an essential skill in nursing, and it helps you to understand the world around you and often to identify how things might be improved. Other activities will help you develop key graduate skills such as your ability to think critically about a topic in order to challenge received wisdom, or your ability to research a topic and find appropriate information and evidence, and to be able to make decisions using that evidence in situations that are often difficult and time pressured. Communication and working as part of a team are core to all nursing practice, and some activities will ask you to carry out teamwork activities or think about your communication skills to help develop these. Finally, as a registered nurse you will be expected to lead and manage your own team, caseload or area of care, and to support junior student nurses in their learning and so some activities focus on helping you build confidence in doing this.

All the activities require you to take a break from reading the text, think through the issues presented and carry out some independent study, possibly using the internet. Where appropriate, there are sample answers presented at the end of each chapter, and these will help you to more fully understand your own reflections and independent study. Remember, academic study will always require independent work; attending lectures will never be enough to be successful on your programme, and these activities will help to deepen your knowledge and understanding of the issues under scrutiny and give you practice at working on your own.

You might want to think about completing these activities as part of your personal development plan (PDP) or portfolio. After completing the activity write it up in your PDP or portfolio in a section devoted to that particular skill, then look back over time to see how far you are developing. You can also do more of the activities for a key skill that you have identified a weakness in, which will help build your skill and confidence in this area.

The challenges of communication seem to persist against a context of globalisation and the continuous movement of diverse individuals and groups of people who require a more robust and intentional approach to their communication needs. Some of these have emerged from the 2020 pandemic and global issues such as climate change, Black Lives Matter, the current economic crisis and instability in the provision of healthcare both nationally and globally.

The authors hope that you find the book a helpful and accessible addition to your learning and an essential tool to help develop and improve your skills of communication in your workplace, your educational environment and your everyday life.

We hope you enjoy the book, and we wish you all the very best with your studies and throughout your career.

Chapter 1

Understanding and applying communication and interpersonal skills

Naomi Anna Watson

NMC Future Nurse: Standards of Proficiency for Registered Nurses

The following platforms and proficiencies will be covered in this chapter:

Platform 1: Being an accountable professional

1.3 Understand and apply the principles of courage, transparency, and the professional duty of candour, recognising and reporting any situations, behaviours or errors that could result in poor care outcomes.

1.11 Communicate effectively using a range of skills and strategies with colleagues and people at all stages of life and with a range of mental, physical, cognitive and behavioural health challenges (Annexe A.)

Platform 4: Providing and evaluating care

4.3 Demonstrate knowledge, communication and relationship management skills required to provide people, families and carers with accurate information that meets their needs before, during and after a range of interventions (Annexe A.)

Chapter aims

After reading this chapter, you will be able to:

- understand communication principles and their personal application;
- communicate confidently with your peers as a means of building a supportive network;
- outline definitions of communication and consider the theoretical perspective;
- explore communication concepts such as the Johari window in the context of individual understandings and application in everyday clinical practice;

(Continued)

(Continued)

- define emotional intelligence, self-awareness and interpersonal skills;
- explore the impact of digital technologies on communication patterns and modern-day healthcare practice;
- recognise potential barriers to successful communication.

Introduction

Communicating effectively is an essential skill for all nurses and healthcare professionals. It underpins the important requirement of ensuring that information is transmitted at a level that meets the needs and expectations of all participants for whom it is intended. For example, using language that is clear and simple, instead of using jargon or acronyms, is one way to ensure that a message is understood. This is particularly important for nurses who work in an environment where there is technical and medical terminology. Patients, carers and their families who are anxious and worried will look to you and your colleagues and supervisors to help them understand what they are being told. If this is done appropriately, it has the potential of adding value not only in clinical practice but in everyday personal life.

In this chapter you will explore some of the principles of communication in the context of your own personal and professional development and consider theoretical perspectives that underpin their application. You'll then explore the Johari window and consider what you may learn from it and identify its relevance to you as a practitioner and how it relates to your self-awareness and interpersonal skills. You get to explore the impact of digital technologies and social media on communications generally and on your communication style specifically. There will also be the opportunity to explore the likely barriers to successful interpersonal communication.

Defining communication

At its most basic level, communication begins with a sender and a receiver and involves the use of verbal or non-verbal cues. Nordquist (2021) agrees that in order to ensure that the message being relayed is not misunderstood, the sender has a responsibility to ensure clarity at all stages of the process. In a twenty-first-century global community, with increasing population migration and advancing digital and technological methods, communication has become complex and sometimes unclear, as we've seen through the rise of so-called 'fake news', for example (Neuwirth et al., 2021).

For you as a student nurse, it's important to remember that good communication begins from an interpersonal perspective. In other words, with you as a person and as a professional at the centre. It may be written, spoken, face to face, or at a distance through digital media such as Facebook, X (Twitter), Instagram or other social media outlets.

You are ultimately responsible for what you say, write, tweet or post. Because of your duties as a public sector worker, you are also governed by your professional body, which expects you to understand the implications for providing quality care that is of the highest standard possible (NMC, 2018). Consequently, communication is an important skill that must be developed and practised for your professional context and growth. This may not always be easy, given the likely difficulties of navigating new environments as a healthcare student, additionally complicated by events such as a global pandemic or other national or international crisis. However, it is an important requirement as part of your professional duty to ensure that you remain self-aware and constantly seek out ways to communicate more effectively as a professional person.

The Department of Health and Social Care (2010) defines communication within a healthcare context as a meaningful exchange occurring between two people aimed at conveying information that may be factual, opinion, feelings thought, which can be either verbal or non-verbal, written or face to face. In the activity below, you will get an opportunity to think some more about your own way of communicating interpersonally with peers and your understanding of this.

Activity 1.1   Communication

1.   Make a list of likely reasons why you will need to communicate with your student peers.
2.   Identify the types of communication you use, whether written, verbal, non-verbal, social media, etc.
3.   Which of these are you most confident with?
4.   Discuss your thoughts with one or more of your student peers and share comparative ideas that you may be able to refer to in your developmental portfolio.

As this is based on your own observation there is no outline answer. However, there is a brief comment at the end of the chapter.

Communicating interpersonally with your student peers is an effective way of practising this important skill. In terms of your introduction to the practice of healthcare and expectations that may be required of you, talking with and to your peers can usually be a safe way to begin to make sense of what is required of you in your role. It gives you the opportunity to share any challenging experiences from clinical practice in a confidential way. It also gives you the chance to reflect on your actions so that you can learn from them, modify your actions and move forward with confidence as you continue to prepare for successful practice (Gibbs, 2013).

To start a process of peer-to-peer communication, an essential requirement is that you introduce yourself to your fellow students if you do not already know them. Introductory details may at times appear to be taken for granted, however, this is an essential early requirement at all levels of communication and is particularly relevant within a healthcare context. So, having ensured that you have appropriately introduced yourself by stating your name, your current role and why you are here, you have access to a supportive network from your peers while providing the same. You get to practise your interpersonal skills on your peers, and you can share and reflect on any challenging experiences, expectations and fears confidentially. You get and give support to each other, and you can compare your thoughts from your learning and prepare for the clinical environment. The important issue to be reminded of in this context is to be mindful of confidentiality, as required by your professional regulatory body, and ensure that people and places referred to cannot be identified (NMC, 2018).

This initial approach to your learning should never be taken for granted as it holds the potential for ensuring that your approaching presence in an active clinical environment can begin in a positive way. It sets the scene for your preparation to approach and interact with patients, carers and other healthcare professionals. Healthcare environments can at times be stressful and difficult. Your best preparation to enter them is recognition of the importance of the introduction in the workplace. Introducing yourself to your peers, patients, their carers and other healthcare professionals is a fundamental underpinning factor in good interpersonal skills, which, surprisingly, is not always evident in healthcare professionals' interactions with patients (Grainger, 2013: Department of Health and Social Care, 2010).

To summarise, peer-to-peer communication provides the following benefits as outlined in Figure 1.1.

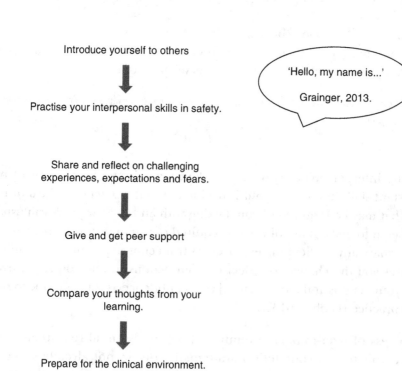

Figure 1.1 Peer-to-peer communication process

Exploring communication theory

An understanding of theoretical concepts helps you to apply your learning to your practice. You can use evidence-based approaches that will improve the way you deliver care to patients and their families. It also helps to improve the way you interact with the multidisciplinary workforce that make up the team in all healthcare settings, whether this is the NHS, or the private sector. Theoretical concepts underpin a better understanding of the different types of interpersonal communication. Norman (2019) identifies four main frameworks that are at the heart of the communication process and summarises the approaches that are available, as follows:

- mechanistic: involving telecommunications using the transmission mode;
- psychological: which has its focus in personal emotional feelings;
- social constructionist: based on how different realities are perceived by individuals from experiences that may be similar;
- systemic: which places communication as one aspect of a whole systems approach that can be revisited and remodelled in separate parts as required.

In the clinical environment, it will be possible to identify any of the above at different points in practice, depending on varied episodes of patient care, or when interacting with different practitioners.

Case study: Riaz

One day, you overhear a conversation between your supervisor and Sarah Lane, a social worker, about Riaz, a 25-year-old patient who lives with autism. His discharge has had to be postponed following his operation to remove his appendix. Your supervisor reports Riaz as being very upset because no one had talked to him about going home. They had arranged everything with his family and assumed that he wanted to go back to his family home, with his parents, however, Riaz had arranged to go and to stay with his best friend Ali, and to then try and find a flat for himself. Sarah Lane said she had assumed that Riaz would want to go to his parents' home.

Activity 1.2   Reflection

- What issues can you pick out from this case study?
- What are the assumptions that have been made?
- Which of the above frameworks did you identify in the interaction?

There is an outline answer to these questions at the end of the chapter.

An important way of strengthening your communication skills is to improve your level of personal self-awareness. This involves the development of a more insightful relationship and understanding of yourself and other people. Goleman (2009) identified specific defining features that can help individuals to focus on self-awareness building. These include your emotional self or your own feelings (and how they influence the way you think and behave) and your personal needs. These are usually identified as a number of psychological factors that tend to impact on the way we behave. Maslow's 'hierarchy of needs' is well known and identifies issues such as basic needs for food and safety and self-esteem, the need for love, affection and self-actualisation (Maslow, 1970). Our individual habits in response to these needs may be automatic actions that form part of our everyday lives, our values and our personality. Alternatively, these can become deliberate actions that drive those responses. Our values and beliefs are also key factors that drive our daily actions. Other defining features of personal self-awareness include your habits, emotions and values. Habits often tend to be actions that happen automatically and may be routinely repeated. An awareness of their likely negative impact on our interactions may help us to modify our behaviours by taking deliberate action.

The best way of building self-awareness includes making a systematic and consistent effort to ringfence time to reflect on what your strengths are, and on the areas of development that may be required including your aspirations and how these can be realised. Reflection is also helpful when working in a therapeutic environment as it provides an opportunity for you to learn from your own actions, including in likely crisis events that may happen in the clinical environment.

The benefits of this include being able to identify likely subconscious aspects and patterns of thinking that may be influencing your behaviours and actions. You can then plan deliberate actions that will help you to modify and improve them.

Psychologists Luft and Ingham (1955) developed a simple psychological tool to enable individuals to gain a better understanding of themselves and others. Their model acts as a method of disclosure with feedback, where individuals disclose aspects of themselves that may not be known, and receive feedback from others, as illustrated below:

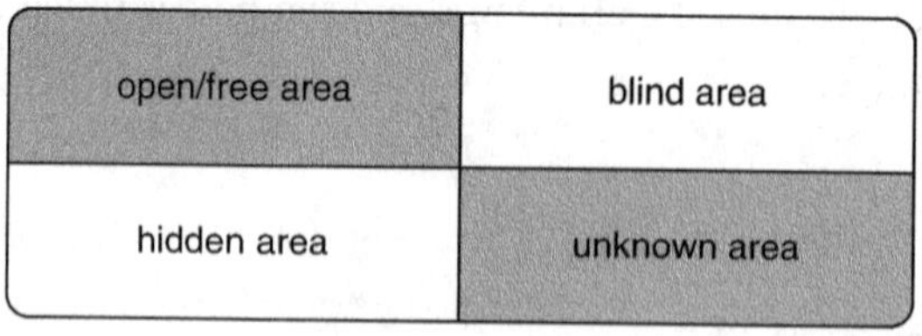

| open/free area | blind area |
| hidden area | unknown area |

Figure 1.2 The Johari Window

(Adapted from Luft and Ingham 1955)

The above tool can be easily and effectively used to help individuals and groups identify and learn how their actions are perceived by others. This is an activity that you can do with your peers.

Activity 1.3   Reflection

1.   Working with a partner or in a small group, make a disclosure and receive feedback on each aspect of the four windows in Figure 1.2.
2.   Share with your peers one thing that you learned from the activity.
3.   Identify anything that surprised you about the feedback from your peers.

As this is based on your own reflection, there is no outline answer.

Emotional intelligence: impact on interpersonal communication

An understanding of emotional intelligence (EI) is another key factor that can positively contribute to the way we communicate with patients and their families and carers. Cherry et al. (2020) define EI as a skill, where one is able to exercise control over, evaluate and have clear perceptions of one's emotions while also understanding the emotions of other people. This then enables the individual to manage people effectively. However, Goleman (2009) argues that EI is a type of intelligence that is positively linked to adults with secure attachments while those with insecure styles, who have high anxiety levels, are negatively associated. Attachment theory is mainly based on the work of John Bowlby (2012) who identified four attachment styles common in adults, as follows:

1.   anxious and preoccupied;

2.   avoidant and dismissive;

3.   disorganised, fearful and avoidant;

4.   secure.

These attachments are developed in early life, based on relationships with significant others such as parents and other caregivers, and tend to form the basis of adult behaviours. A secure attachment style is linked to strong, positive bonds with primary caregivers, where a child develops expectations about people and the world based on the ways that their own needs were met during childhood.

The major critical concerns in research on EI are whether it is innate, or present at birth, or whether it is all learned. However, what has clearly emerged is that those who have a high level of EI appear to be able to perform better at their jobs, have strong leadership skills and are able to sustain better mental health and wellbeing (Segal, 1997).

The mixed model

Goleman (2009) also identified a mixed model of EI as follows:

Table 1.1 Goleman's mixed model

Self-awareness	having the ability to understand one's strengths, weaknesses, emotions, goals and values, and recognise how these may impact other people. This then helps to guide decision-making
Self-regulation	self-regulation or being able to redirect and control all emotions that may be disruptive by adapting to situations that are changing
Social skill	being able to regulate personal relationships and get along with others
Empathy	having the ability to consider the feelings of others before making decisions about them.
Motivation	having a clear understanding of what drives individual behaviour

Goleman also discussed emotional competencies which are not necessarily linked to intelligence but are learned behaviours, which can be developed and improved with education. This is despite his theory that generic EI is present at birth, with which there is some disagreement in the literature (Segal, 1997). The mixed model incorporates skills and values that are important specifically when working as a nurse. Most are embedded in your code of conduct (NMC, 2018) and are expected behaviours when interacting with patients in the clinical environment.

Case study: Lisa

It is Lisa's first day on the medical ward and she is accompanying her supervisor on the medication round. They arrived at the bedside of 48-year-old David Hines, a cardiac patient, to give him his medication. Lisa called his name and waited for a response but noticed that he did not reply. On checking closer, and trying to wake him up, her supervisor noted that David had collapsed and was not responding to stimuli. She instructed Lisa to lock the medication trolley, pull the curtains and bring the emergency trolley to the patient's bed, while she pressed the button to call the resuscitation team. Lisa was not sure where to find the emergency trolley and while she was frantically looking for it, a full team of people arrived and someone else brought the trolley to the bedside. David Hines did not recover despite receiving resuscitation treatment from the emergency team. Lisa was very upset about the incident and was not happy when, later that morning, she was also asked to accompany her supervisor to perform last offices for David. She had never done this before.

Activity 1.4   Reflection

Thinking about Lisa's case study, how do you think EI may have impacted on Lisa's and her supervisor's response, if at all?

What could have been done differently if anything?

There is an outline answer to these questions at the end of the chapter.

An individual has to be able to manage their emotions and it is worthwhile remembering that EI can be affected by stressful situations.

Digital technologies and likely impact on communication

The information superhighway has brought with it not only opportunities, but challenges for the nursing profession. As a student, you will no doubt have been exposed to the myriad of digital technologies that now exist, not only in your personal life, but also in your student capacity. In this section we explore digital technologies and their likely impact on your student experience.

Although there has been a move to introduce the use of technology in NHS healthcare, some have argued that this has not kept pace with the rapid developments in the sector (RCN, 2022b). You would have by now encountered a number of technological aids and may have had an opportunity to engage with them with your clinical supervisors. The computer is now a standard addition to most clinical environments, but the research suggests that systems are not always as efficient as they ought to be, and instead of providing the best support for nursing care and positive patient outcomes, instead, they sometimes slow down clinical activities because of the length of time they take to load information (Robichaux et al., 2019).

Throughout the Covid-19 pandemic digital and verbal platforms of communication between multidisciplinary teams (MDT) were the predominant means of communication. This shift was unexpected and swift, with immediate necessary changes required in order to extend the adoption of technology across healthcare sectors specifically in the NHS. As a consequence, a rapid digital transformation is underway in most if not all healthcare settings. It is now time to analyse the use of digital technology and its actual impact on the experiences and safety of patients. Additionally, the effects on student and staff experiences in terms of the time to care, will now need to be explored.

Activity 1.5   Observation

Arrange with your clinical supervisor to participate in or observe a digital consultation with a patient. You'll need to ensure you gain the patient's permission. Make a brief summary of how and where the consultation was done, the supervisor's introduction and interaction with the patient, the outcome of the consultation, documentation shared, closure and total timings.

- How did you feel about how the session was conducted?
- Was anything missing?
- How could it be enhanced?

As this activity is based on your own observation, there is no outline answer.

The Royal College of Nursing (RCN, 2022) offers a range of top tips to enable practitioners and patients to have a positive experience when undertaking digital consultations. Suggestions include the following:

- Introduction: say who you are and what your role is.
- Establish the identity of the person you are speaking to.
- Ensure the environment is quiet and private and that the patient can hear and understand.
- If a patient appears to be struggling to understand or to communicate, find out if there is anyone else available that may be able to help.
- Make reasonable adjustments for disability, English as a second language, neurodiversity, cognitive impairment or hearing difficulties. Services such as language line may be helpful. Using family members to interpret must be used with caution due to poor interpretation or sensitivity when discussing certain issues, for example with children.
- Respect patients' rights to refuse to discuss certain topics at all times. They should be reassured that they can change their minds and be given information to contact clinical staff when/if they decide to do so.
- Ensure records and documentations are accurately kept to reflect what was discussed. You should include that the consultation was remote.
- Check if a chaperone will be required and arrange as appropriate.
- Check understanding and agree any further actions that may be required. Document patient responses and reinforce any agreed forward actions.
- Arrange a follow-up if required. Ensure the patient understands how this will happen and keep a record of this.

Digital awareness, digital poverty and patient care

The times they are a changing

(Neuwirth et al., 2021, page 141)

The digital age has introduced a variety of enhancements to the way patient care is planned, organised and delivered. Being able to engage and interact with patients and support them with any devices that they may be using as a part of their care is now an essential aspect of care planning. Whether it is on a ward, or in the community, you will need to be aware of the possibilities of having to develop and expand your digital awareness in order to provide effective care and advise and support carers and families.

Digital awareness also involves developing an understanding of possible digital poverty, which was exposed by the Covid-19 pandemic when many UK families were forced to work and school from home together. The strain on technology availability was a major factor influencing families' abilities to support their children effectively while also working and needing to use the one major device available to the household. The response of healthcare providers and professionals has the potential to contribute to enabling patients and service users and their carers to quickly grasp the benefits of harnessing new technology to support their health. It also helps early recognition of likely problems so that solutions can be found as quickly as possible (Hutchings, 2020). This is in order to acknowledge that there is no going back, the digital age has arrived for good. It is now up to society and government to ensure that there is equity of access in order to reduce digital poverty, especially during a time of austerity and impending global recession that the UK also currently faces.

Scenario: Jeremy

As a student in your second year of study, you are on placement in the community and have been assigned to your supervisor Mavis, who is the district nurse leading the team in the health centre. On your second morning in the clinic, she invited you to sit in on a consultation she was having with Jeremy, an 18-year-old patient who has type 2 diabetes. Jeremy was telling your supervisor that he was interested in using a digital gadget he had heard about, called the Freestyle Libre System to help him monitor his diabetes a little more effectively as he was tired of sticking a needle in his fingers. He wanted some more information about it. Your supervisor was not sure about this gadget and asked you whether you had heard about it. You recall having to study this topic on your course and had done some research about it for a project.

Activity 1.6   Communication

Discuss all the different ways that you could communicate and share this information with Jeremy as the patient, Mavis as your supervisor and all the other members of the team in the clinic.

There is an outline answer to this question at the end of the chapter.

Within a nursing perspective, the Digital Capacity Framework (2015) identifies six domains that are considered to be important to enable and strengthen digital understanding and use as part of nursing skills, values and behaviour. As a student, you are in an ideal position to develop and expand your learning in this area, and to contribute to workplace innovations and developments that will improve patient care. The domains are listed here for you to consider their application personally and in practice.

1. digital identity, wellbeing and safety;
2. communication, collaboration and participation;
3. teaching, learning and self-development;
4. technical proficiency;
5. information data and media literacies;
6. digital creations, innovation and scholarship.

Activity 1.7   Communication

Using numbers one and two of the six domains, make notes based on your past experience of using digital media. Talk about any advantages you have gained from using the media as a student nurse, and any problems you experienced. Then visit the Digital Capacity Framework website (see 'Useful websites' at the end of chapter) and compare the information provided there.

As this activity is based on your own experience, there is no outline answer.

The need for all nurses to be able to effectively manage their online presence and identities both personally and professionally, is widely emphasised in the literature (Topel, 2019). This includes being able to manage your own time online in an effective way and being able to spot and respond to online abuse and bullying. There is also a requirement to support your peers and your patients to help them manage their online presence safely and effectively. This is particularly important in the case of children and young people, who may be influenced by negative exposure to online content and come to harm as a result. Additionally, all online content posted becomes quickly public, is easily copied and circulated, and may affect your ability to get employment as a nurse, or you may have to face disciplinary processes if it is not appropriate. It's vital that you don't share details about patients unless this is done in a confidential manner so that patients cannot be identified from your discussions. You should also not share personal details about yourself and family unless it is safe to do so.

Your understanding of digital technologies is an essential aspect of delivering care in the twenty-first century. Patients of all ages and walks of life now own a digital 'gadget' and are willing to use it to support their wellbeing. For example, utilising their mobile phone to help them manage their illness or fitness has become a regular feature of self-care, and as a student nurse or a qualified practitioner, you should be able to encourage all your patients to participate in this activity.

Potential barriers to successful communication

Being aware of likely barriers to your communication is an important requirement while working in the clinical environment. This awareness will help you to think about the issues and seek to find ways of overcoming them when interacting with patients, their families, carers and other professionals that you have to work with (Watson, 2019). Working in the health service will bring you in to contact with a diverse group of people that includes patients and healthcare workers from around the world and from different contexts and cultures. Barriers to successful communication are, however, also possible even among those with whom you identify socially and culturally. They could be caused by an illness or other condition affecting a particular service user. Carter (2019, page 85) noted some factors that could become potential barriers and create communication vulnerability. Examples include intrinsic factors such as a visual or hearing impairment, dementia, cerebrovascular accident (CVA) or a stroke, cancers of the head and neck, traumatic brain injury or progressive neurological conditions such as Parkinson's disease, multiple sclerosis, or motor neurone disease.

Extrinsic factors include the physical environment such as noise, acoustics, lighting, written information, culture, language, perceptions of healthcare professionals and level of support for family and carer. While these will all be issues that we may have no control over, raising your personal awareness will drive the ability to adapt and adjust as necessary to improve and enhance communication in each of the areas identified.

Case study: Adam Green

Adam Green is 65 years old. He is a father of two grown children who are both married and live away from home. He lives with his wife. Adam had a CVA which left him with speech and language difficulties and the loss of movement on one side of his body. Jane, the student nurse, was assigned along with her supervisor, Susan, to care for Adam while he was an inpatient on the ward. Adam became frustrated and angry at being unable to express himself to his carers and to his wife Sally. He was lashing out at staff and had become difficult during caring encounters. His two children who used to visit, stopped coming because they said they were fed up with his behaviour and anger towards them and their mum. Sally complained to the staff that her husband was being difficult and was taking out his frustrations on her. She was at her wits end with this problem and didn't know what else to do. She feared that she was no longer able to cope and asked Jane's supervisor in her presence what else she could do to make life easier for her husband before he returns home. He was due to go home in a week's time and Sally said she was dreading it.

Activity 1.8   Communication

1. Identify the barriers that are affecting all parties in the caring encounter in the Adam Green case study.
2. What can Jane, as a student, and her clinical supervisor do to support Adam and reduce his frustrations about making himself understood and support interactions between him and the staff who care for him?
3. How can Jane support his wife and children through this difficult time?

There is an outline answer to these questions at the end of the chapter.

As you consider the many likely barriers that could negatively affect communication, remember to also stay aware of personal extrinsic barriers that could impact on the way you interact in clinical practice. As Carter (2019) suggests, your own perceptions as a healthcare professional may also act as a barrier if not appropriately managed. The influences on this can be many and varied, and include culture, language use and the physical environment. To enable successful interactions, it is important to plan communication encounters appropriately.

Activity 1.9 Reflection

Make a list of your own extrinsic personal barriers that could impact on the way you communicate. Think about issues such as language, culture and attitude.

- What steps can you take to address the impact on your relationship with your patients and your supervisor, and the medical and other professional staff?
- When you get an opportunity, book a 15-minute tutorial session, and ask your supervisor about extrinsic barriers to communication and which ones they think are relevant to you in your current practice.

As this activity is based on your own reflection, there is no outline answer.

Chapter summary

In this chapter we have considered some of the main principles and theory of communication. We have explored definitions and peer communication in the context of Granger's (2013) theory, looked at self-awareness and the Johari window and explored emotional awareness and intelligence and their implications for patient care. We've also identified how digital technologies, digital communication, the internet and social media may influence your practice as a nurse and how to mitigate their risks. You will now be able to apply these important principles to your practice and begin to contribute to enhancing the care of patients and their families. Additionally, you have gained insights into the way you communicate with your peers, lecturers and supervisors which should enable a better learning experience.

Finally, we discussed communication barriers that may result from a variety of causes such as intrinsic factors including supporting a patient and family with a CVA and extrinsic factors relating to personal perceptions of healthcare professionals.

It is imperative that you take ownership of your communication skills development and work towards ensuring that your patients receive high-quality care as a direct positive outcome from your own knowledge, understanding and experience of the digital information superhighway.

Activities: brief outline answers

Activity 1.1 Communication (page 9)

You should have been able to identify a number of reasons why you will need to communicate with fellow students.

You can get, and give support from each other by sharing resources, etc.

You might be part of a social network support group on a platform such as WhatsApp, with other student peers, so you can call or message them, or meet up with them face to face to discuss a topic or even to just socialise.

Some people are not confident with group chats, social media channels, or with speaking up on online forums. This may be something to think about in terms of how you manage it for yourself and others.

You can write down your feelings about these issues and talk to your peers or even your supervisor, about the best ways to manage communication encounters.

Activity 1.2   Reflection (page 11)

It is clear that Riaz was not consulted about his wishes for discharge. The arrangements had been made with his family. Assumptions may have been made based on the fact that Riaz lives with autism, that he should go to his family home, perhaps his family had also assumed that he should come home to recover. However, Riaz wanted to use the opportunity to leave home, and he had a practical plan in place to do so.

Aspects of the psychological and social constructionist framework emerge here, with Riaz getting upset that, at age 25, and an adult, no one had asked him about his wishes. Both your supervisor and Sarah Lane, who had made the arrangements, had also assumed that this was acceptable to Riaz.

Activity 1.3   Reflection (page 13)

A ward emergency such as the unexpected collapse of a patient can be a stressful event to deal with, especially if you are new to that environment. The incident is one that both Lisa and her supervisor may find useful on reflection to consider what they could have done differently. Lisa can also think about why she is unhappy to perform last offices for David and will need to be given time to process the events of her very first day on the cardiac unit. How Lisa manages her EI following this incident is likely to determine her eventual responses as a student nurse and as a future qualified practitioner.

Activity 1.6   Communication (page 17)

You have a number of options available to you as a student to choose from to share information. As you are in a meeting with a patient and have been invited to comment, you may want to quickly give a brief overview to your supervisor and patient, of what you know about the gadget. You could offer to follow up with more information by sharing a website or writing details about the Freestyle Libre Device (see 'Useful websites' below). If you know anyone who uses one, you may also be able to find out if they would be prepared to come along and share their experience of its use, and invite the patient to attend, at a later date.

Additionally, as a student, you could ask your supervisor for permission to prepare and run a development session for everyone in the clinic about digital gadgets or specifically the Freestyle Libre. This could then include a learning pack or a poster that could be placed in the staff education centre. The above activities would give you the opportunity to develop a range of communication skills that will enhance your personal and professional development.

Activity 1.8   Communication (page 19)

It is clear that Adam's frustration with his limited ability to make himself understood is affecting him negatively. There will also be some frustrations with regard to you and your supervisor. However, as his carers, you may both be more familiar with the likely impact of a stroke on patient behaviours.

There are many ways to support Adam. You could use basic charts with simple 'yes' or 'no' responses. You could ask him to nod or shake his head if he is able, to signal a positive or negative response. Jane and their family will need support from you and your supervisor to help them through this difficult time. Referral to NHS talking therapies, and other relevant members of the multidisciplinary team (MDT) will be a good place to start. Active listening skills are essential to ensure that their concerns are heard, and actions taken to respond to their needs.

Further reading

Digital NHS (2017) Health Survey for England, 2016. Available at: digital.nhs.uk/data-and-information/publications/statistical/health-survey-for-england/health-survey-for-england-2016 (Accessed: 12 August 2022).

Comprehensive information about the NHS digital strategy for moving forward.

Health Education England (HEE) (2017) A Health and Care Digital Capabilities Framework. Available at: rcn.org.uk/-/media/royal-college-of-nursing/documents/clinical-topics/a-health-and-care-digital-capabilities-framework.pdf (Accessed: 27 November 2023).

A very useful document that gives a clear summary of HEE's plans for moving digital capability forward.

RCN (Royal College of Nursing) (2017) Improving Digital Literacy. Available at: www.rcn.org.uk/Professional-Development/publications/pub-006129 (Accessed: 27 November 2023).

Provides insights into ways of extending and improving digital literacy among nurses.

Useful websites

www.freestyle.abbott/uk-en/home.html

This website provides useful details about the Freestyle product for patients who live with diabetes.

www.jisc.ac.uk/building-digital-capability

The Digital Capacity Framework website with details on building digital capability

https://portal.e-lfh.org.uk/

The NHS England e-learning resource for healthcare.

Chapter 2 Communication and power relationships

Kay Norman

NMC Future Nurse: Standards of Proficiency for Registered Nurses

The following platforms and proficiencies will be covered in this chapter:

Platform 6: Improving safety and quality of care

6.2 Understand the relationship between safe staffing levels, appropriate skills mix, safety, and quality of care, recognising risks to public protection and quality of care, escalating concerns appropriately.

Platform 7: Coordinating care

7.1 Understand and apply the principles of partnership, collaboration, and interagency working across all relevant sectors.

7.13 Demonstrate an understanding of the importance of exercising political awareness throughout their career, to maximise the influence and effect of registered nursing on quality of care, patient safety and cost effectiveness.

Chapter aims

After reading this chapter, you will be able to:

- demonstrate awareness of how health policy influences nursing and consider your own role in 'speaking up';
- understand how assigned and perceived power can affect communication in collaborative working;
- identify situations where escalation is needed in practice, including whistleblowing, and communication strategies you might use.

Introduction

Helen Donnelly, a registered nurse, collected her OBE in 2014. She was recognised for raising concerns about care at Mid-Staffordshire NHS Foundation Trust and supporting her colleagues to do the same to protect patient safety. Helen subsequently worked as an ambassador for cultural change at the Staffordshire and Stoke on Trent Partnership NHS Trust. She was seen as a role model for other nurses to challenge poor care and encourage whistleblowing, helping to launch NMC guidance on raising concerns for nurses and midwives. The Mid-Staffordshire NHS Foundation Trust inquiry in 2013 now seems in the distant past, but it is important to learn from past experiences to reflect and improve. Thankfully, recommendations from this report continue to be realised, but it is important for nurses to take responsibility for coordination of care and feel able to challenge and raise concerns in a well-informed, constructive way. Not every nurse will receive an OBE or become a recognised ambassador, but every nurse should be politically aware and recognise how they can influence healthcare services in coordinating care for patients. Identifying and escalating concerns can be challenging as a student nurse, but it is essential to understand your responsibility in this aspect of patient and public safety.

This chapter introduces the concept of power in developing, improving and challenging relationships through effective communication. You will explore your own perceptions of what you see as the role of the nurse and other health professionals in coordinating care in a changing political landscape. You will reflect on how these influences may impact you as a student nurse when working with patients as partners, and how the communication strategies you use can help to facilitate organisational change and raise concerns appropriately.

The history of the present

To understand the present, we must learn from the past. D'Antonio (2006) suggests that the promotion of historical awareness in nursing can help the profession to build resilience, critical thinking and a strong professional identity. The terms health and illness are socially constructed in different communities around the world, with the term 'medicalisation of health' being particularly prevalent in Western cultures. Until the 1800s most illnesses were managed by family members or someone (mainly women) within their community who had a reputation as a healer. In contrast, historical archives show the role of a physician, although unregulated at this point, was fulfilled by men to treat rich families who could pay for treatment.

During the pre-First World War period of 1881–1914 nurses were recruited based on 'caring' traits and those who were not interested in marriage or children, dedicating their lives to their vocation. The growth of hospitals towards the end of the nineteenth century as a result of increased industrialisation saw government social control in helping to limit the impact of illness for workers. This can be seen as the first state involvement in health. Medicine and healthcare saw a shift away from the traditional religious and pastoral origins towards a more scientific arena.

Medicine was subsequently seen as a highly skilled profession with nurses assisting doctors in promoting recovery from illness/surgery. Medicine developed a strong voice as a profession and as a political influencer. Nursing has slowly developed a professional identity and with the existence of the Nursing and Midwifery Council (previously the United Kingdom Central Council), is now a recognised and regulated profession. Nevertheless, we can see from the nursing discourse that power and equal status with other health professions has been historically difficult to harness in influencing change (Holme, 2015). Government bodies, such as the National Health Service (NHS) and Department of Health and Social Care will ultimately dictate health policy and priorities.

Case study: Government influences on healthcare during the Covid-19 pandemic

During the recent Covid-19 pandemic, Public Health England (PHE) produced regular guidance and updates on how health professionals should be managing and treating patients with Covid-19 symptoms and also how to protect the public with a mass vaccination programme. Hospitals and healthcare providers were receiving regular notifications to update policies and processes to reflect government strategy and guidance. This was a new experience for global healthcare and countries around the world adopted various approaches, with the World Health Organization producing principles and guidance. Vaccination clinics were implemented to ensure the UK population were appropriately protected. Face-to-face GP appointments were suspended as was visiting relatives in hospitals and care organisations. Most routine surgery was cancelled. The NMC introduced a temporary register to encourage nurses back into practice. Healthcare professionals were seen as heroes and the public diligently clapped weekly on their doorsteps for NHS workers. Government proposed a mandatory vaccination programme for all healthcare workers and healthcare organisations set about navigating the complexities of terminating or suspending employment contracts for those who refused vaccination. A hospital doctor refused to agree to this mandate, which was broadcast as part of a visit from the then health secretary to his place of work. It transpired that many key personnel were refusing to be vaccinated so the decision for mandatory vaccination was overturned.

Activity 2.1   Critical thinking

- What communication methods were employed to influence vaccination uptake?
- How do you think positions of power influenced the decisions made in this scenario?

As this activity is based on your own observation, there is no outline answer.

The global pandemic required population-based communication strategies to influence uptake of vaccines. Constant media coverage evidencing the devastating mortality rates of Covid-19 alongside daily 5 p.m. news updates from the UK prime minister, credible physicians and public health specialists focused the requirement for everyone in the UK to be vaccinated. Government decisions indicated who would be first to receive these. The messaging included promoting a sense of 'duty' to be vaccinated to protect loved ones and others, and specifically mandated for key workers. Nevertheless, it has been demonstrated that government policy can be affected by other influencers, such as professional organisations and unions, and decisions subsequently overturned.

How professions are portrayed through varying communication methods will continue to influence perceptions of nursing. Consider the imagery of nurses and other health professionals and where you have seen these images. This could include news items, television documentaries, social media posts, books and magazines, YouTube videos, or even fancy-dress parties. Take a moment to reflect on how they have affected your perceptions of nursing.

Your own communication of what 'nursing is' can leave a lasting impression on friends, family and also your colleagues. These networks may ultimately become users of a healthcare service and remember your views. The NMC Code (2018) contains professional standards which must be upheld. One of these standards is to 'promote professionalism and trust', which helps guide your responsibilities. You will see this standard applied in clinical practice and learn from a range of role models that will help you navigate and understand these concepts. Discussing nursing situations and how you feel is encouraged in your learning. This will help to identify what went well and what didn't go so well in order to understand and improve. However, you must be mindful of how this could affect others and consider who and when you communicate. From the discussion above, we can see it can be difficult to navigate your responsibilities to promote change when there are historical barriers to overcome. Cultural change within healthcare continues, and you should be proud to be part of influencing that change.

Activity 2.2   Critical thinking

The following two aspects of the NMC Code relate to the above standard 'promote professionalism and trust':

20.7 Make sure you do not express your personal beliefs (including political, religious, or moral beliefs) to people in an inappropriate way.

20.10 Use all forms of spoken, written and digital communication (including social media and networking sites) responsibly.

- In what ways could the above affect how you talk about nursing to others?
- What do you think 'inappropriate' and 'responsibly' means in this context?

As this activity is based on your own observation, there is no outline answer.

This activity will increase your awareness of the NMC Code and how terms can be mis-interpreted. It will also encourage you to think about what these terms mean to you personally and professionally. Communicating responsibly might mean different things to different people so it is important to explore this further with your practice assessor/practice supervisor or university lecturer.

The concept of power in healthcare relationships

The concept of power has been briefly discussed above in terms of history, health policy and government influences. Power can be authorised by virtue of an assigned role. For example, a ward manager can be assigned authority to manage staff, services, and ultimately have responsibility for decision-making at a certain corporate level. A nurse or student nurse may also be seen as being in a position of power by demonstrating expert knowledge to plan and care effectively for their patients. Power can be used constructively to 'do good' but you might experience situations where power, authorised or perceived, is used destructively. It is important for all health professionals to work together to provide the best standards of care possible. This relies heavily on effective communication and respect for each other's roles and viewpoints (Brooks, 2018). We can draw on experiences where it may have been difficult to question people with assigned power, such as a teacher or manager. As a student nurse it may feel as though everyone in your allocated practice area has more knowledge and expertise than you, which makes them seem 'powerful', including those who presume they have power but do not have assigned authority. It can feel difficult to challenge any position of power, assigned or otherwise. Understanding various communication strategies can help to overcome possible feelings of fear and anxiety.

As a student nurse starting a placement experience, you want to 'fit in' with the team and make the most of your learning experience. Building effective relationships is paramount to achieving this (see Chapter 5). You will draw on your experiences from other areas and will have built some understanding of what an effective team is, with all members being respectful of each other and listening to others' viewpoints to work collaboratively, no matter what role is assigned within the team. Braithwaite et al. (2016) discusses multidisciplinary teamwork (MDT) where groups of professions tend to demonstrate tribalistic tendencies in the workplace and conform to stereotypes. Their research suggests that taking health professionals outside of the workplace demonstrates effective MDT and therefore concludes that workplace culture is responsible for individuals conforming to stereotypes. You may see aspects of this in your placement experiences and reflect on your own professional socialisation into nursing. Your practice assessors (PA) and practice supervisors (PS) will help shape your learning experience throughout your student journey, demonstrating the values, behaviours and standards required to instil positive professional socialisation (Norman, 2015). Drawing on positive role models and discussing concerns with your PA/PS or university tutor can help you navigate and learn from these experiences.

Scenario: Team working in a GP surgery

Imagine your placement allocation is within a GP surgery. You are working with the practice nurse during an asthma clinic when a child becomes wheezy, and the mother becomes extremely anxious and distressed. The practice nurse, who is an independent prescriber, commences to use a nebuliser on the child and asks you to fetch the doctor to examine them. The GP enters the room, examines the child, and prescribes steroids. He does not speak with the child, mother or practice nurse and returns to his surgery clinic. The practice nurse comments that he is a poor communicator but a great doctor. You witness several occasions where the GP ignores staff, does not acknowledge patients, you, or the practice nurse during the working day, but this is accepted as the norm.

Activity 2.3   Communication

Looking at the above scenario:

- How might this particular GP's communication style affect the culture of the GP surgery? Why do you think this is accepted?
- What communication styles could be effective in challenging this behaviour?

There is an outline answer to these questions at the end of the chapter.

When behaviours, attitudes and poor communication are not challenged, they become part of the accepted culture and are normalised. The more extreme consequences of this can be seen in news items leaving people feeling shocked at the standard of care being provided, with healthcare teams accepting their colleagues' poor behaviour. A BBC *Panorama* programme in September 2022 highlighted repeated instances of poor care, neglect and abuse within a large hospital providing care for patients with mental health and learning disability needs in Manchester (*Panorama* team and Joseph Lee, 2022). Registered and non-registered healthcare professionals were seen abusing vulnerable patients, with their colleagues ignoring this behaviour.

Challenging authority constructively

Drawing on Pajakoski et al.'s (2021) integrative literature review, it is seen as essential that nurses demonstrate moral courage to promote patient safety. This concept is well researched with a growing body of knowledge evident in nursing, psychology and philosophy. Nurses with moral courage are seen to be willing to take personal risks to protect patient care, overcoming any fear to ensure high standards of nursing care are achieved. Moral courage also requires admittance of mistakes to others and learning from these to improve. As a student nurse, you will begin to develop moral courage through experience, knowledge and competence. Confidence is needed to be morally courageous and as a student nurse you will need to seek support from your placement organisation and education programme/university staff. Hierarchy in organisations can affect and inhibit moral courage, with nurses acknowledging difficulty in being courageous if they need to challenge someone higher in the professional group (Kleemola et al., 2020). The most important thing to ask yourself is *What could happen if I don't speak out?*.

As discussed above, the NMC Code provides standards of professional behaviour to guide our practice. Ultimately, nurses want to care for their patients in the best way possible, however, everyone will experience periods of personal challenge, stress, anxiety and illness at some point. Working in a collaborative team will acknowledge this, with colleagues willing to support each other through varying complexities. There may be occasions where a member of staff will appear agitated and rude in their response if they feel under pressure. Consider what might have elicited the response. No one should feel bullied or upset during a clinical placement experience, although taking time to reflect on someone's poor communication can help to understand possible reasons for this. For example, was the individual particularly rushed/busy, were they completing a complex activity which required focus and concentration, were they tired? Did they realise they were rude in their response? Often during busy clinical activity, poor communication responses are not recognised by the individual. It is important to be honest and constructive, acknowledging your own feelings and the possible reasons that could have affected the communication response (Norman, 2019).

Non-verbal communication methods, such as e-mails, should be used with caution when expressing feelings as misinterpretations can occur. The receiver of the message cannot see your face, body language, or hear the tone of your voice. If in doubt, ask a trusted friend or colleague to read the e-mail out loud and give their opinion. Be respectful in your message and be clear that you value the individual's response. Look at the case study of Mike, a second-year student nurse:

Case study: Mike

Mike was excited to commence his placement at a busy Accident and Emergency Department, however, he felt during his first few days he had not been integrated into the team and did not know who his assigned practice assessor was. Following a very busy night shift, Mike sent the following e-mail from his mobile phone before going home.

Dear Julie

I am e-mailing to let you know I am not happy with my learning experience. Your staff have not completed my initial interview yet and I haven't met with my practice assessor. I have just completed my fourth night shift in your department, so this is unacceptable. I am going to let the university know too. I have been working with healthcare assistants and practice supervisors but have not had an opportunity to complete any proficiencies. Can you let me know when I will meet with my assessor as soon as possible?

Mike (student nurse)

Activity 2.4   Communication

How could an e-mail be constructively worded to foster respectful communication and receive a positive outcome?

There is an outline answer at the end of the chapter.

In the case of Mike above, the recipient of the e-mail may feel the tone of the e-mail is aggressive, and this might affect their response. It is important that Mike's learning is protected, and he receives supportive and effective supervision and assessment, although it is also important to recognise the possible pressures and priorities of a clinical working environment at any one time. O'Luanaigh's (2015) research identified that registered nursing staff were aware of their responsibilities as facilitators of learning but acknowledged that barriers such as time constraints, patient priorities, and support for the recognition of their role could impact on achieving this effectively. Taking time to think and reflect on the wider situation can help to construct an e-mail that identifies your concerns, whilst acknowledging aspects that could be influencing the current situation. Never send an e-mail when you are angry, frustrated, or upset until you have taken time to consider how this will be received. Speak with your university tutor or placement link if you feel unable to speak with someone in the clinical practice area. Consider if an e-mail is the most appropriate form of communication to effect change or result in an action. Scheduling a short meeting with the ward manager or nominated person for the practice area to discuss concerns in person can be followed up with an e-mail to clarify discussion points raised and resulting agreed actions.

Remember you are an advocate for patients, and you have a duty to be open and honest, adhering to the NMC Code to raise concerns. Encouraging transparency can facilitate learning, improvement and appropriate action planning for teams and organisations. The following case study relating to Zosia will help you to consider the possible issues that can arise from unplanned situations and how teams can learn from these cases.

Case study: Zosia

Zosia has attended a busy outpatients clinic for assessment of her mental health following several episodes of self-harm and refusing to eat. Zosia has previously expressed suicidal thoughts and is known to the community mental health team. Zosia has attended the clinic with her guardian who is waiting in the clinic reception area. The psychiatric registrar who completes the assessment feels Zosia should be admitted due to safety concerns and the need for further assessment. The registrar informs the nurse manager that the patient must not be left alone. He takes Zosia's notes with him to arrange admission but has to first see another patient. The ward manager asks a third-year nursing student to stay with

Zosia until they can arrange admission to a ward. Another patient is creating a disturbance at the reception area using abusive language and shouting at staff. A staff nurse asks the student nurse to call security urgently while she tries to defuse the situation. The student nurse can't remember the number for security given during her induction, so she calls the main reception number, which takes some time to answer. Security arrives after 15 minutes. During this time Zosia has left the consultation room and cannot be found within the outpatients clinic. Zosia's guardian is still waiting in the main reception area.

Activity 2.5   Critical thinking

- What communication errors occurred in this case?
- Should this be reported as an adverse incident and, if so, who is responsible for reporting?

There is an outline answer to these questions at the end of the chapter.

Unplanned and adverse situations do occur within all care environments despite effective communication, good team working and shared decision-making. Patient safety is paramount, so when things go wrong it is necessary to report all instances. As a student nurse you will not normally be required to report mistakes or near misses to the patient or carer involved, nor submit a report to the organisation or relevant regulators, however, you will be expected to support team members in this activity by recalling facts and initiate the concern if necessary. All healthcare organisations will have a policy for reporting adverse incidents and you should also follow your university guidance.

Raising concerns and whistleblowing

At the beginning of this chapter, we referenced the Mid-Staffordshire inquiry where a nurse had courage to raise concerns about the poor care and poor organisational management she witnessed within one NHS trust. You may have seen other media stories that provide harrowing accounts of mismanagement and poor care within healthcare environments. One of NHS England's (2012) 6Cs is 'courage' but this can often be difficult to demonstrate for the various reasons discussed above.

Since the Mid-Staffordshire NHS Foundation Trust Public Inquiry (Francis, 2013), healthcare organisations have ensured policies relating to raising concerns and whistleblowing are embedded within their services. Speak-up guardians are named individuals for any member of the healthcare team to contact if they have any concerns. It is important to understand that there is a difference between raising concerns and whistleblowing. The law sets out these differences and identifies six specific criteria which must be met for raising concerns to qualify as whistleblowing:

- *The person raising the concern is a 'worker' – someone who works or worked under a contract. This extends beyond formal contracts of employment and includes employees, agency workers, trainees, volunteers, student nurses and student midwives.*
- *The person raising the concern must believe they are acting in the public interest. This means that a number of people stand to benefit if action is taken on the concern, and it is not solely for personal gain. Personal grievances and complaints are therefore not usually whistleblowing.*
- *The person raising the concern must believe that it shows past, present or likely future wrongdoing in one or more of the following categories:*

    o *that a criminal offence has been committed, is being committed or is likely to be committed.*

    o *that a person has failed, is failing or is likely to fail to comply with a legal obligation;*

    o *that a miscarriage of justice has occurred, is occurring or is likely to occur;*

    o *that the health or safety of any individual has been, is being or is likely to be endangered;*

    o *that the environment has been, is being or is likely to be damaged;*

    o *that information showing one or more of these criteria has been, is being or is likely to be deliberately concealed.*

- *The person raising the concern must believe that the matter falls within our regulatory remit.*
- *The person raising the concern must believe that the information they disclose is true.*
- *In raising the concern, the individual must not themselves be committing an offence.*

(NMC, 2022)

Whistleblowing can take place within the organisation, or if the person does not feel able to do this, they can raise it with a third person known as a 'prescribed person'. The NMC is named as a 'prescribed person' in law.

You should be informed of the raising concerns and whistleblowing policies for the placement organisation within the first few days of commencing your clinical learning experience. If this is not communicated to you, ask your PA, PS or nominated person to direct you to these policies. Your university will also have their own processes for students raising concerns in clinical practice. It is important to understand these, what is expected, and the actions you should take. All care staff should be working to reinforce these policies and encourage and support each other to identify poor practice. If you are unsure whether to raise a concern, speak with someone who can help you reflect on what you have observed and discuss how to take your concern forward. This could be your tutor, PA/PS, nominated person, or clinical manager. In most instances, organisations will be grateful that you have identified a concern. Some issues can be actioned quickly with an appropriate action plan developed to monitor progress. If things don't feel right, always ask the question *Why am I feeling this way?* It is better to communicate how you are feeling about a situation than to ignore it. The case study below is an example of how actions can be implemented effectively if concerns are raised.

Case study: Raising a concern in practice

Aaliyah, a first-year student nurse, was enjoying her clinical placement. During her first few weeks, she had witnessed patient call bells not being answered, even though staff were sitting talking at the nursing station. Aaliyah, healthcare assistants and other students seemed to be the only ones answering these call bells and registered staff would only help when asked which meant there was a significant delay in all call bells being answered. Aaliyah spoke with some of the more senior students and asked how they felt about the situation. Two third-year students agreed it was poor practice, but they did not want to raise it as an issue, as their final proficiencies needed to be signed off in this placement. They agreed to raise it at their university practice evaluation day. Aaliyah felt this wasn't right so reviewed the university policy for raising concerns and contacted her personal tutor. Aaliyah's tutor thanked her for having the courage to raise this and contacted the nominated person in placement. All students in this placement were subsequently asked to share their experiences. A meeting was held with the interim ward manager who immediately ordered a call-bell monitoring audit. The manager discussed the issues raised in a full team meeting with all staff and students, giving everyone the opportunity to voice their opinion. The meeting focused on patient care and professionalism, including the importance of all staff and students feeling able to question any practice they observed in order to improve nursing care. All staff were asked to offer reasons for the non-answering of call bells, possible solutions, and interim goals, which helped to formulate an initial action plan that would be reviewed in four weeks. Named call-bell monitors were appointed for every shift. Registered staff reflected on their professionalism and role modelling, acknowledging the concern raised and committed to improving their practice. Aaliyah thought she would be isolated for raising the concern but all those involved assured her she had done the right thing.

Activity 2.6   Reflection

Reflect on the case study above.

- Do you think Aaliyah communicated her concerns effectively?
- Would you have done anything different?
- How do you think Aaliyah should be supported?

As this activity is based on your own observation, there is no outline answer.

'You said, we did' is a phrase that is becoming increasingly popular to communicate actions from issues raised. Speak with your university tutor to understand how this works for your course. Finding the courage to raise a concern is admirable and experiences of the process should be shared. Awareness of your student services support in addition to your own personal support networks can be helpful to offer advice and signposting to relevant agencies.

The above case study provides an example of a positive outcome from raising a concern, although we know from previous studies that it is not always an easy process. Jack et al.'s (2021) research provides student nurse narratives of their reporting of poor care. Although aspects of challenging behaviours proved difficult, resulting in some upset students and angry registered nurses, students were prepared to speak out to improve patient safety, overcoming their fear of bullying and isolation to protect patients. Communication strategies varied including immediate verbal challenging of the registrant's decision-making 'in the moment', questioning the care activity 'in the moment', and accessing other health professionals for support following the event. Team culture has been identified as a strong influencer in whether student nurses will raise a concern in practice (Fisher and Kieman, 2019).

Encouraging open, transparent learning environments can support questioning of practice and welcoming ideas for improvement. Students who are made to feel part of the team where their voices can be heard and acknowledged can help to overcome a perceived status of low position in the nursing hierarchy.

As you move towards registration as a nurse, you will be part of the next generation of leaders and role models. Foster an open communication culture to support organisational policy to raise concerns. Reimagining how raising concerns can help and improve practice, rather than displaying defensive behaviours in continuing with the status quo, can encourage healthcare teams to remain patient centred at all times.

Chapter summary

This chapter has provided an insight into how communication can be used and affected by assigned, perceived and assumed power in relationships. It has highlighted scenarios to consider in terms of how you might respond in a similar encounter and reflect on your own understanding of your role as a student nurse in the multidisciplinary team. The chapter has discussed your responsibilities in raising concerns and how this can be communicated effectively.

Activities: brief outline answers

Activity 2.3 Communication (page 28)

An individual who does not engage in effective communication with team members can affect the culture and behaviours of the whole team. In this scenario, no one questioned the GP's behaviour as it was accepted as normal. This could be due to their position of assigned power in the organisation. Nevertheless, failure to communicate with team members and patients can impact relationships, potentially causing misunderstandings, fear and treatment errors. Transparent and open conversations are inhibited and learning opportunities as a team are missed.

Communication strategies to address this could include:

As a student nurse, discuss this with your PA/PS. Previous history might be useful to help understand the current communication situation.

Develop written ground rules for team meetings so all staff feel able to constructively challenge each other to improve patient care.

Involve all staff in discussing the benefits and disadvantages of effective communication in a safe meeting space.

Present relevant communication case studies as learning opportunities.

Your PA/PS could support speaking with the GP during a quiet time, acknowledging the GP is extremely competent in their role but asking if they are okay. Discuss how important it is that the team work together and highlight recent positive examples of this. Give an example of how their communication has made you/members of the team/patients feel and ask if they were aware of this. In many instances, the individual may not be aware of how their behaviour is affecting others.

Activity 2.4 Communication (page 30)

Good morning Julie,

I hope this e-mail finds you well.

By way of introduction, I am a second-year student nurse and have been looking forward to my learning experience in the Accident and Emergency Department. During my first four night shifts this week I observed a range of nursing care activities and going forward I want to ensure my learning plan reflects the range of opportunities available.

I wanted to highlight to you that I've not met my practice assessor yet, so I would really appreciate if you could let me know details of who has been allocated to this role. I can then make contact to arrange a meeting as soon as possible to discuss my goals and proficiency requirements during this clinical placement, as required by the university. I do appreciate how busy this department is and would like to feel part of the team over the coming weeks. I have attached a brief plan of actions I can take to encourage this so I would welcome your thoughts.

I look forward to hearing from you.

Kind regards

Mike Davies (second-year student nurse)

Activity 2.5 Critical thinking (page 31)

This case study highlights the potential for significant harm to a patient and therefore should be viewed as a near miss/adverse incident. Members of staff involved in this scenario might discuss and agree who will escalate this, but it is important that it is reported as soon as possible after the event via the organisation risk management system or relevant policy/procedure.

When a situation is reported as an adverse incident, it is important that learning from the event is discussed and shared with all members of staff and patients/carers involved, and also wider members of the team to reduce the risk of this happening again and improve patient safety. Staff should be supported throughout subsequent discussions to ensure a 'no blame' culture is promoted.

We can see from this case study that staff did not communicate effectively. The psychiatric registrar informed the ward manager that Zosia should not be left alone but failed to give the rationale for this request or details of her case. He had taken Zosia's notes with him to arrange admission, so no one was able to view his written records. The ward manager allocated a student nurse to sit with Zosia, but no explanation was given as to why this action was needed or the importance of not leaving Zosia alone. Zosia's guardian did not receive any communication from staff and was not informed of the care management proposed. The department team were not alerted to the situation that resulted in a staff nurse asking the student nurse to leave Zosia and call security. There was a delay in security responding as the student nurse had not memorised the organisation's emergency call number during her placement induction. The student nurse did not call out to staff to ask for the emergency number and continued to wait for the main reception switchboard to answer.

Further reading

Arnold, E and Underman Boggs, K (2022) *Interpersonal Relationships: Professional Communication Skills for Nurses*, eighth edition. Missouri: Elsevier.

This resource will provide you with additional discussion and case studies relating to interpersonal relationships during episodes of communication activity. Chapter 9 in particular will help you understand self-concept in the context of professional interpersonal relationships.

Brown, P, Jones, A and Davies, J (2020) Shall I Tell My Mentor? Exploring the Mentor–Student Relationship and Its Impact on Students Raising Concerns on Clinical Placement. *Journal of Clinical Nursing*, 29(17–18): 3298–3310.

This article will help you reflect on the student experiences presented in these research findings. You will gain an awareness of the challenges that can be faced when raising concerns and your responsibility to overcome these to protect patients.

Lukes, S (2021) *Power: A Radical View*, third edition. London: Macmillan Publishing – Red Globe Press.

This is a classic book which explores power as a concept within social and political theory. This will help you understand how power conflicts can affect personal and organisational communication activity.

Useful websites

assets.publishing.service.gov.uk/government/uploads/system/uploads/attachment_data/file/279124/0947.pdf

Report of the Mid-Staffordshire NHS Foundation Trust Public Inquiry: Executive summary HC 947, session 2012–2013. This report is useful background to read. It evidences numerous communication errors and highlights genuine fear of staff in challenging authority.

nmc.org.uk/standards/guidance/social-media-guidance/read-social-media-guidance-online/

Social media guidance: The Nursing and Midwifery Council. This guidance will support your understanding of regulatory requirements for using social media in practice.

nmc.org.uk/standards/guidance/the-professional-duty-of-candour/

The professional duty of candour – the Nursing and Midwifery Council. This joint guidance from the NMC and General Medical Council (GMC) includes reporting accidents and near misses, the responsibility to inform necessary organisations and regulators, and being honest with the patient.

nmc.org.uk/standards/guidance/raising-concerns-guidance-for-nurses-and-midwives/whistleblowing/

An overview of NMC guidance to whistleblowing and your responsibilities as a student nurse.

nmc.org.uk/education/becoming-a-nurse-midwife-nursing-associate/raising-concerns-as-a-student/

These case studies provide an opportunity to reflect on your understanding of what went wrong and what could have been done differently.

Chapter 3

Communication in different settings

Naomi Anna Watson

NMC Future Nurse: Standards of Proficiency for Registered Nurses

The following platforms and proficiencies will be covered in this chapter:

Platform 1: Being an accountable professional

1.2 Understand and apply relevant regulatory and governance requirements, policies, and ethical frameworks including mandatory reporting duties, to areas of practice, differentiating where appropriate, between the devolved legislatures of the United Kingdom.

1.18 Demonstrate the knowledge and confidence to contribute effectively and proactively in an Interdisciplinary team.

Platform 2: Promoting health and preventing ill health

2.4 Identify and use all opportunities making reasonable adjustments when required, to discuss the impact of smoking, substance and alcohol use, sexual behaviours, diet and exercise on mental, physical and behavioural health and wellbeing, in the context of people's individual circumstances.

Platform 4: Providing and evaluating care

4.8 Demonstrate the knowledge and skills required to identify and initiate appropriate interventions to support people with commonly encountered symptoms including anxiety, confusion, discomfort and pain.

4.15 Demonstrate the knowledge, skills and confidence required to provide first aid procedures and basic life support.

Annexe A: Communication and relationship management skills

2.5 Identify the need for and manage a range of alternative communication techniques.

Introduction

There are a wide variety of settings in the community where care is delivered to those who need it. People perhaps immediately think about the hospital, which has over the years tended to be the focal point of care for those who are sick. However, most people usually begin to experience symptoms of illness in their own homes, and with the onset of a recent pandemic (Covid-19) when people were unable to go to a GP when they became ill, or could only go to a hospital when they were acutely ill, more and more people are remaining at home where possible, and being cared for by the use of varied digital technologies to support their illnesses (RCN, 2022). This increase in, for example, the video and telephone (telehealth) in the consultative process calls for a high level of communication skills both from medical and nursing staff. Primary care is undergoing rapid changes in a care system that faces many challenges to the way care is delivered to people.

Primary care as home care, versus digital care

Case study: Jennifer Green

Jennifer Green is 75 years old and lives with her husband Ben who is 80 years old and has Alzheimer's disease. Jennifer lives with type 2 diabetes and is the main carer for her husband. Recently she called her GP to complain that she was depressed and exhausted, saying that she is not coping well with caring for Ben. She was asked to attend the surgery, however, she declined and requested a video consultation with her GP. The practice was initially reluctant to arrange this, however, she advised them that she has an iPad, which her grandson had bought her and had shown her how to use. She is comfortable with using the Zoom app, which her grandson has installed on the device for her. The practice arranged a video consultation as requested. The online consultation was attended by Hanifa, a second-year student nurse, and her supervisor Fiona, the general practice nurse on duty that day. Hanifa and Fiona are known to Jennifer and have previously seen her at the diabetic clinic. The meeting lasted for 15 minutes, and Jennifer asked about treatment for her depression and said she was not sleeping well at night. She enquired about support with caring for Ben, and also asked about sleeping tablets. Her GP advised her that he would request Mary, the district nurse, to visit and do an assessment prior to prescribing any medication, but that the visit may not take place for a couple of days due to workloads.

Activity 3.1 Decision-making

1. What do you think are the issues, if any, with this situation?
2. How else could it have been managed?
3. Find out how often the GP practice provides a video consultation and reasons why they do or do not.
4. Find out about the use of virtual ward environments in your region and which GP practices, if any, subscribe to it.

There is an outline answer to these questions at the end of the chapter.

At a time when the use of digital technologies to support nursing and healthcare is being widely encouraged, it is expected that telehealth, which has been in use even before the recent Covid-19 pandemic, will continue to be a main focus for the delivery of care to people in their own homes. Plans to invest and extend the reach of digital and online services in the support of healthcare delivery and practice is clearly outlined (DHSS, 2022). All UK providers of health are expected to engage with this agenda and make intentional efforts to ensure that NHS staff and patients are supported to make the practical application achievable and successful. However, there are always challenges to implementing new systems in NHS care delivery practice, which also have to be understood and a commitment made by all to identify and deal with these. Effective leadership is required but resource availability is also an essential element of any implementation (Karreinen, et al., 2023). From nursing perspectives, guidance to members is also provided by NHS England (2024) to help them with developing and setting up a professional approach to the use of digital technology such as telephone or video conferencing, among other initiatives. Historically though, home care was provided by district nurses in patients' homes, which is still the case today. Continued digital initiatives will need to be embraced and accepted by all staff in order to move care delivery into the new global digital world. A further good example of this initiative is the introduction of 'the virtual ward' which has been a part of NHS remote services in the context of 'hospital at home'. This is a service that is provided virtually by the NHS to provide acute online care to patients in their own homes. It is not difficult to recognise how important the new concept is and its potential to transform the NHS, which suffers from extensive staffing shortages and other resource limitations (O'Malley et al., 2022). Obviously, there are limitations to what can be provided in terms of clinical care remotely, for example where specific clinical procedures such as operations or other hands-on care are required. However, early discharge post operations or other clinical procedures is currently standard procedure in an NHS that is regularly short of beds. The virtual ward could fill an important gap in care provision and ultimately reduce the strain on NHS resources.

Primary healthcare, however, has a wider meaning that encompasses a range of factors discussed below.

Primary healthcare – policy perspectives

Primary care in the UK provides the initial point of contact for patients who need help with their health and wish to access care from the NHS. Historically, The World Health Organization (WHO), in its Alma-Ata Declaration in 1976, paved the way for what was to become the cornerstone of primary care globally. It was considered essential care, underpinned by methods that are not only sound but based on robust scientific evidence. It should be available in the community to people and their families in a cost-effective manner for country and community. It was also considered to be essential to economic and social development in all societies (WHO, 2020c). There were specific nation goals that all countries were expected to commit to fulfil and included:

- the provision of basic sanitation;
- immunisation against major infectious disease;
- prevention and control of local endemic diseases;
- promotion of an adequate supply of safe water;
- adequate nutrition for their nation;
- control and prevention of health problems by education;
- adequate services to include maternal, childcare and family planning services;
- appropriate treatment for common diseases and injury.

At the time of its original inception, the goal of the Alma-Ata Declaration was to achieve health for all by the year 2000. The expectations included the need for health sectors to work with local and national agencies in an attempt to encourage and promote cooperation and trust. This should enable progress to be made in delivering improvement in health where it matters most, at the heart of the community. While major steps in the improvement of primary healthcare globally have been achieved, especially in wealthier countries, the WHO (2020b) still identifies primary care as an area needing continuing emphasis globally to meet the changing nature of the environment and of disease processes. This is especially since the end of the recent Covid-19 pandemic, which was responsible for very high mortality rates globally and identified many gaps in healthcare systems worldwide, but perhaps unexpectedly also in the wealthier healthcare systems of the global north.

The WHO's Alma-Ata Declaration was the key underpinning factor that led to major changes to primary care in the UK. Hence a continuous process of policy and legislative change and development has always been a feature of primary care. From the historic introduction of Primary Care Trusts (PCTs) in the early 1990s to the onset of Clinical Commissioning Groups (CCGs) later on, changes continue to influence the ways services are arranged, funded and delivered in the community. At its most simplistic, the GP might be considered by most to be at the heart of this arrangement, and this may be the case. However, people in the community have had access to other community-based services from the very inception of the NHS, some of which they are required to fund for themselves, for example, ophthalmic services and dental services, to name two. In more recent times, pharmaceutical services have also become much more directly accessible to individuals. Pharmacists are able to provide help and guidance with minor illnesses and prescribe for these if appropriate.

The GP surgery may be located in a community health centre, which is usually shared by a number of GPs and may also provide other health services. The concept of primary care was initially led by an increasingly ageing population demographic with people living longer but not necessarily healthier, bringing with it an increasing likelihood of requiring care. This was identified by the Office for National Statistics (ONS, 2021c) well over a decade ago, as over 95 per cent of people who will eventually need to be cared for in their own homes and communities. The current climate of issues facing the NHS, include low staffing levels, unavailable beds and bed-blocking by older people who may not be acutely ill but need support (RCN, 2022a). This has led to the continuing unsustainability of meeting all these demands in the face of the ever-increasing cost of funding services, hence re-emphasising the importance of primary healthcare services. Providing care at home via 'the virtual ward' that reflects the level of care that may be received in an acute hospital may be considered care that reaches beyond that which is traditionally provided by district nurses (DNs). If you get an opportunity to participate, you will be able to undertake your own evaluation as a student to assess how this service contributes to improving care quality outcomes in the NHS.

Principles of primary healthcare

Primary healthcare is based on principles that specifically identify certain processes in terms of what patients and communities can expect. According to NHS England (2023) These include five pillars that underpin the focus of care delivery and practice in community settings. They include the following:

1. social equity;
2. nationwide coverage;

3. self-reliance;

4. inter-sectorial coordination;

5. people's involvement in planning and implementation of programmes.

These principles form the basis of delivering care and must be reflected in all your actions as a student nurse. Notice how these are reflected in your code of practice (NMC, 2018) and how they align with the WHO's original Alma-Ata Declaration of 1976. Ultimately the end goal of primary healthcare is to shift the emphasis from the disease process to the users of services, the people in all communities. The emphasis is on 'care' rather than 'cure'.

Primary care versus secondary and tertiary care

Providing care in patients' homes

Communication outside of any recognised healthcare setting may be more challenging because there is some shift in the power base. This is true for visits to patients' homes, as it is for having a telephone or video conversation with a patient while they are in their own homes. Patients usually feel less vulnerable when they are at home with their families, and most may have even explored the online technology for themselves so that they are clued up when they have a conversation with a healthcare specialist. Additionally, paper records are usually left in patients' homes. The majority of patients have access to their digital primary care record as promised by NHS England (Davidge et al., 2023). Any paper record is also accessible by patients and their carers and families. It is important then, to be self-aware as a student nurse, and to spend time developing appropriate communication skills for both writing and reporting on patient records. The language used must be written in a manner that will not offend patients and families if they choose to read them, but factual and reflective of actual summary accounts of what was said and what was done. This will enable you to display a high level of professionalism while in conversation with patients in various settings whether this is their home, or another venue in the community. It must be noted that homecare may also be classed as one aspect of primary care services, as patients would have had to make contact with their GP or other provider as a first point of contact, to trigger home visits for the purpose of carrying out nursing care.

Secondary care, on the other hand, is simply care that is being provided following on from a referral either by an individual patient's GP, or another member of the inter-professional or MDT. Usually, the referral is to medical services specialists who do not normally have contact with any patients, except through referral. This chapter gives you the opportunity to think about the way you communicate in varied settings and apply the skills you are learning to enhance the patient experience and improve care quality outcomes in the NHS. Tertiary care on the other hand is usually that which is provided via referral bypassing the patient on to the next suitable care provider. The purpose of all three care systems – primary, secondary and tertiary care – is to ensure a smooth single pathway as an integrated care system. This becomes challenging and perhaps at times confusing when there are historical misunderstandings or unclear trajectory about processes of moving patients on, especially when the terminologies are used to mean different things to different groups of care givers and providers. Examples include terms such as community nursing, district nursing, community care and home care, terms that many use with varied meanings (Watson, 2001). Care in the community has tended to be slightly misunderstood especially as it initially related to the historical closing of institutional care establishments for people with learning disabilities. In community practice, this is an enduring problem, which means that caregivers and care providers need to be aware of this and ensure that there is clear common understanding when each term is being used in practice.

Consider the scenario below as you begin to explore ways of communicating while providing nursing care in someone's home.

Scenario: Care provision in a patient's home

You are a second-year student nurse on your first community placement with John, the district nurse who will be your supervisor for the duration of your placement. You arrive at the health centre on your first day on duty in the community and set out with John to visit a patient's home. He informs you that he has a full caseload that day, starting with a leg ulcer dressing for a lady who is expecting an early visit. You arrive and John introduces you as his new student to Mrs Mary Brown who has leg ulcers on both lower legs, with dressings on. John starts to prepare the new dressing set, so, to be helpful, you proceed to remove the outer dressings, placing them on the floor. However, Mrs Brown refuses to let you remove the second layer of her dressings saying that her legs are very painful to touch, and John is more used to taking them off. Moreover, she says, you have not washed your hands and she doesn't want them to get infected. John takes over from you and begins to talk to you about the procedure for removing a dressing, including what to do with it once it's been removed. You are a little upset as you were only trying to be helpful.

Activity 3.2   Reflection

1. Identify the issues in this care delivery experience for you as a new student nurse in the community environment, and for the patient.
2. What could both you and your supervisor have done differently?
3. How do you think this experience will influence your future practice?

There is an outline answer to these questions at the end of the chapter.

Preparation for any placement, especially one in a different setting from a hospital ward, requires being able to effectively communicate by taking the initiative, where possible to ask your supervisor questions about the placement, the requirements and what may be expected of you. Being proactive and checking things out prior to starting this placement carries the benefit of ensuring that you are informed and reduces the risk of awkward incidents in the patient's home or even in the health centre. As on the hospital ward, there are specific protocols when delivering care in a patient's home. These will help to embed good practice in your delivery of any subsequent care. For example:

- You must be invited into the patient's home, so always knock, even if the door is open and they are expecting you.
- Do not place your treatment bag on the floor, even if the floor looks clean enough: this is not good practice.
- Ask the patient's permission to place your treatment bag somewhere clean and safe, for example on a nearby table or sturdy clean chair.
- Ask permission to wash your hands and ask where you can do this.
- Alternatively, if you have antibacterial hand rub that you have travelled with, you may use this, once you have placed your treatment bag somewhere clean and safe. Be sure to make it clear that you are cleaning your hands prior to commencing a care procedure. Patients will be taking note of specific hygiene issues so never take it for granted.
- Ask for privacy if this is required for the treatment you are carrying out, and there are other people in the room. This could reduce distraction and save some time.
- Once again, wash your hands, or use your antibacterial hand rub prior to completing paper records of care.
- Request the paper patient records from the patient if applicable, so you can first read earlier entries of other staff prior to starting any care procedures.
- Ask permission from the patient prior to starting and carrying out any treatment.

The establishment of CCGs in 2012, the most recent change in services, was an important policy change, brought about as part of the Health and Social Care Act published in 2012 (Legislation.gov.uk, 2012). In 2013, CCGs replaced PCTs, however, in July 2022, as a result of the new Health and Social Care Act of 2022 (Legislation.gov.uk, 2022), CCGs were closed down and integrated care systems (ICS) were legally established to place emphasis on inter-sectorial coordination. Organisations are required to work together so that future planning of services can reach its ultimate goal of providing as seamless a care as possible. ICS has two specific statutory aspects, an integrated care partnership (ICP) and an integrated care board (ICB). Their goal is to come together locally to plan and pay for services. Local partnerships include public sector services, local councils, the voluntary sector and local people. Their specific objective is to ensure that care provision meets local care needs, is of a high quality and is affordable. The new changes should contribute to better access, more joined up care and improvement in care quality outcomes. Devolved care in all UK nations is largely modelled on the structure in England, however, each has specific aspects that are peculiar to the nation concerned. For example, some services that are free in one country may not be available for free in another. These can be explored further from a nationwide perspective via the links in the 'Useful websites' section.

Emergency care
The Accident and Emergency (A&E) Department

Here you get an opportunity to consider the issues that influence care in UK A&E Departments. This environment is considered to be one of the most stressful sections of the NHS in which to practice. The majority of A&E Departments have traditionally busy times, usually reflective of weekends when most people may be off work and have decided to enjoy their time off with excessive use of alcohol or engaging in sports activities that may cause injury. The usual outcome is a trip to A&E usually because of an accident or other mishap on their way home from a party or public house. A lot of effort has been made to reduce the inappropriate use of A&E. This has the potential to save on costs (Ismael, 2013). However, patients know that they can enter as walk-in patients and may not always use other services such as the 111 service or the urgent care service. The case below, though, is an example of appropriate use and highlights other issues that are likely in this environment.

Case study: David's heart attack

David Winterburn is 65 years old and lives with his wife Jill. Their daughter Sonia lives out of town and tries to visit with the grandchildren on a monthly basis.

David became ill one day while he was at home with Jill. He felt very nauseated and began to have intense chest pains which made him breathless, cold and sweaty. The pains were so intense that Jill called the ambulance service (999). It arrived 25 minutes later, and David was taken to the A&E Department, which was half an hour from where they lived. Because he was in pain, and struggling to breathe, David was seen immediately on arrival by a member of the triage team who assessed his condition and ensured that he was seen by a doctor immediately. He had been given oxygen therapy by the ambulance team. Following his electrocardiogram (ECG), the doctors confirmed that David had suffered a massive heart attack. He was given emergency treatment in A&E, but because of bed shortages he had to wait in the A&E Department for 15 hours, before he could be transferred to the Coronary Care Unit (CCU) for further treatment and observations. Sonia, their daughter, arrived some time later and wanted to know what had happened.

Jill was very upset and told Sonia she was unsure about his treatment. She also said that he had been left for a long time on an uncomfortable trolley. They were not happy with this. They both wanted further explanation. The doctor tried to explain, however, after the doctor left Jill and Sonia requested further explanations from the charge nurse Timothy, saying they did not understand what was happening. Timothy was supervising Jane, the student nurse, that day.

In the case of David, the decision to call the ambulance so they could get him to the A&E Department was sensible. He had suffered a severe heart attack, and it was imperative that he was seen as soon as possible. A cardiac arrest requires treatment immediately, or as soon as possible. Without expert help, David may have died.

The decision to attend A&E must be carefully made. NHS England (2022) advises that calling an ambulance should only be done if an individual is unable to breathe, has collapsed, or is facing a life-threatening problem. This is to ensure that services are available to those who need it since resources can sometimes be limited. In England, waiting time in A&E can be as much as four hours. Times may vary in other nations and regions of the UK, but there are a range of other illnesses that can be covered in other environments such as urgent care centres and walk-in centres.

The decision to choose an urgent care centre rather than A&E is not always an easy one for the public. However, there are regular media campaigns reminding people that they can first ring 111 for advice about the best place to turn up. In the case of a suspected cardiac incident, patients are always advised to ring 999 immediately.

Patients can still make a personal decision about where to turn up, and they will not be refused treatment. The key message is that where an illness is considered to be life-threatening the A&E Department should always be the first point of patient access.

Minor injuries and walk-in centres

Scenario: Care in a walk-in centre

You are spending time in a minor-injuries unit and walk-in centre in a busy city centre. The centre treats high numbers of patients who are refugees and as it is close to a university, many international students also regularly use it. There are some challenges with communication.

Lateef, a 25-year-old refugee patient from Pakistan, tried to explain his symptoms using terminology that was vague and unclear. You ask your supervisor if you could have an interpreter to help. Your supervisor advises you that the centre is unable to fund an interpreter so you will have to manage without one. Lateef kept asking for the doctor as he did not understand you either.

Activity 3.4   Communication

In the absence of an interpreter, what other steps can you take to communicate with those who struggle with fluency in English?

There is an outline answer to this question at the end of the chapter.

It is important to note that walk-in centres can help with a wide range of problems including some urgent issues too. Patients also need to be advised that a doctor and other suitably qualified professionals are usually present so they can be reassured about their care. Some members of the public may mistakenly consider the A&E to be the only place where a doctor is available, which makes it the place of choice on account of that 'fact'. Education of the public is important to promote uptake of the service. If a presenting problem is outside of the skills of the team, patients should be reassured that they will be referred on as appropriate. Communication is once again the key ingredient and making sure that the message is understood by all patients is vital.

Nursing people in different settings: roles and responsibilities

Your main responsibility is to be alert and aware of the need to modify the way you communicate with patients, their carers and families in any environment. In an age of digital technology, this does involve being much more conscious of your attitudes especially towards those about whom assumptions can very easily be made that could exclude them from participating in technological advances that could improve their access and utilisation of care in any environment or setting. Specifically older people should be encouraged where possible, to engage with these advances and supported to do so at all times.

Chapter summary

In this chapter, you explored primary, secondary and tertiary care and their relevance in the community. You considered how primary care is delivered and organised.

You explored the policy perspectives and looked at the importance of effective communication using different methods. You identified the varied settings in which people are cared for in the community referencing accident and emergency settings, urgent care environments, the virtual ward and remote digital contexts and some likely factors that affect care in these environments.

This should provide you with a clearer understanding of how care is delivered in alternative settings and help you to become more familiar with ways that you can adapt your skills of communication according to what is required in the workplace.

Activities: brief outline answers

Activity 3.1   Decision-making (page 39)

It appears that the surgery may have been reluctant to offer a video appointment because the patient is an older person. Make sure that this is not the case. However, since the system of tel-ehealth was used throughout the pandemic when people were unable to attend, GP surgeries should be able to offer this alternative consultation to all who request one. Additionally, NHS has a digital strategy that includes various ideas relevant to bringing a variety of digital service methods and practices to patient level.

In line with appointment availability, when Jennifer telephoned to book the appointment, perhaps a district nurse visit could have also been arranged either for the same day or the day after.

Further details about the virtual ward concept are included in the further reading section, but finding out from your supervisor about its practical feasibility and whether your region subscribes is a good learning outcome for you as a student nurse.

Activity 3.2   Reflection (page 43)

Your first day in a patient's home as a student nurse is always a daunting one for most, even with your supervisor. You are on the patient's territory and are a guest in their home. Preparing for the visit is a good idea so that it can go as smoothly as possible. It may have helped to contact your supervisor prior to arriving to ask about the placement and what to expect. It may have also been useful to ask John and the patient first if you can do anything to help. As we said, you are in the patient's home as a guest. Asking her permission before you start any procedure is very important.

A planned introduction to the placement would have been a very good idea, however, with large caseloads and booked visits, with patients waiting, at times district nurses are not always able to spend the required time to help students settle in. Perhaps a telephone call prior to starting, or even making prior arrangements for a visit to the base to meet with staff and get a personal overview may have helped. The main lesson here is the importance of understanding that including the patient in care outcomes does mean asking their permission to carry out procedures. This applies in different settings, such as the patient's home, as it does in an acute hospital ward.

Activity 3.3   Critical thinking (page 46)

As a student, and in the first instance, you may not feel confident enough to answer relatives' queries about a life-threatening illness. However, you need to be aware that patients and their families look to you for support and guidance in times of crisis. You should be able to immediately reassure the family that David is being looked after by skilled professionals and that as soon as a doctor is free, they will be able to explain further.

You will also be working with a supervisor to whom you can go for help and support if you are unsure about what to say. If you are new to the A&E Department, you may want to ensure that as soon as you get an opportunity, you can begin to do some research about cardiac disease and cardiac arrest. The emergency environment can at times be very busy, however, you should still be able to schedule some time with your clinical supervisor and ask some questions about the condition to help you become more confident when dealing with patients and families.

Services in different regions of the UK may not always be at the same level. Once you have talked to your clinical supervisor in your region, you can also check the website of either one or all the other regions when you have the time to do so or have a conversation with your peers to discuss similarities and differences.

Activity 3.4   Communication (page 47)

Based on the environment, the ideal situation would be to have an available telephone online interpreting service, however, you have been told by your supervisor that this is not available.

- Your immediate need is to be able to understand the patient. Since you are in a university community with many students attending, it may be possible to find out if anyone present may be able to help. You could take the lead and suggest this to your supervisor, and while it is not an ideal situation, it may fill an immediate gap. You may take this a step further by suggesting to your supervisor that an approach to the local university could be made for any student studying languages, for example.
- You could also use illustrative drawings to show and get a response from the patient if it is possible to prepare these, or some could be prepared beforehand with basic general images that patients can point to. Since you are in the community, you could arrange to have a 10- or 15-minute tutorial with your supervisor about interpreting services in such settings to explore how you both may be able to advocate for such a service.

Further reading

McCullough, K, Andrew, L, Genoni, A, Dunham, M, Whitehead, L, Porock, D (2023) An Examination of Primary Health Care Nursing Service Evaluation Using the Donabedian Model: A Systematic Review. *Research in Nursing and Health*, 46 (1): 159–176.

A research-based article which uses a systematic review to explore and evaluate primary healthcare services using the Donabedian model (2005), a tool used by the NHS to evaluate and measure quality of care.

Sellman, D (2011) *What Makes a Good Nurse – Why the Virtues Are Important for Nursing*. London: Jessica Kingsley Publishers.

This is a very helpful book which identifies and discusses the core values and virtues of nursing and provides an excellent resource for reading and reflecting on your practice in the context of these essential values.

Useful websites

www.gov.scot/policies/primary-care-services/

Provides services to people in Scotland.

primarycareni.co.uk/

Provides services to the people of Northern Ireland.

nwssp.nhs.wales/ourservices/primary-care-services/

Services provided for the people of Wales.

pcse.england.nhs.uk/

These services are specific to England. However, NHS England serves as the basis for devolved care to the other countries in the UK.

www.nuffieldtrust.org.uk/news-item/virtual-wards-the-lessons-so-far-and-future-priorities

Discusses the virtual ward initiative and looks at its future potential to improve safe access to remote care services.

www.publichealthnotes.com/primary-health-care-phc-history-principles-pillars-elements-challenges/

Provides information about primary care principles and pillars for practice.

www.england.nhs.uk/commissioning/who-commissions-nhs-services/ccg-ics/

Gives a good overview of the structure and purposes.

Chapter 4

Communication in the context of 'race' and cultural competence

Naomi Anna Watson

NMC Future Nurse: Standards of Proficiency for Registered Nurses

The following platforms and proficiencies will be covered in this chapter:

Platform 1: Being an accountable professional

1.14 Provide and promote non-discriminatory, person-centred and sensitive care at all times, reflecting on people's values and beliefs, diverse backgrounds, cultural characteristics, language requirements, needs and preferences, taking account of any need for adjustments.

1.19 Act as an ambassador, upholding the reputation of their profession and promoting public confidence in nursing, health and care services.

Platform 6: Improving safety and quality of care

6.5 Demonstrate the ability to undertake risk assessments in a range of care settings, using a range of contemporary assessment and improvement tools:

6.8 Demonstrate an understanding of how to identify, report and critically reflect on near misses, critical incidents, major incidents and serious adverse events in order to learn from them and influence their future practice.

Annexe A: Communication and relationship management skills

1.5 Use caring conversation techniques.

1.7 Be aware of own unconscious bias in communication encounters.

1.12 Recognise the need for and facilitate access to interpreter services and material.

Chapter aims

After reading this chapter, you will be able to:

- discuss communication in the context of 'race', historic aspects, current issues and likely implication;
- explore cultural competence and its application to clinical practice in terms of sociocultural factors;
- explain unconscious bias and sociocultural factors that influence and underpin interethnic interactions;
- understand the importance of intersectionality, social justice and antiracist healthcare practice, and their likely impact on health inequalities;
- identify ways to address diversity in communication issues in nursing and healthcare through diversity championing, and implications for improving patient satisfaction and care quality outcomes.

Introduction

In the current social and community structures in the UK, all who provide health and nursing care in clinical practice will, at some point, be caring for patients who are from minority ethnic communities. While their presence may be in a minority on wards and in hospitals in some parts of the country, person-centred care that will meet individuals' specific needs must be provided. There is evidence that this care is being compromised in terms of access, inclusion and care delivery practices (Raleigh and Holmes, 2021, Watson, 2001, 2019). A consequence of this is that the quality and safety of care they receive as individuals is questionable.

In this chapter, you get an opportunity to explore the issues, examine the implications, discuss and reflect on ways of improving your communication skills in clinical practice in the context of race and cultural competence. The choice of race as an area of exploration highlights current issues relating to care experiences of minority ethnic people that have contributed to poor outcomes in terms of quality of, and access to care. Some of these will be discussed here by way of illustration and to encourage reflection on how you care for these patients, including likely perceptions that may influence your practice and the practice of your peers and colleagues. Race for the purpose of this chapter is defined by Hartigan (2010) as a system that is used to classify people into groups with the added ranking of those groups implicitly or explicitly in terms of superiority or inferiority. So, race as a system indicates that the concept is socially constructed. This structural process underpins the positioning of minority ethnic people that has led to their racialisation and to subsequent acts of racism against them. Implicit within this is the imposition of otherness, which contributes to keeping 'them' different. Smith (2008) contends that motivational ignorance is a contributor to racism, suggesting the notion that there is likely to be some level of intentional ignorance, or lack of knowledge involved at some point. However, others argue the opposite, stating that an avoidance of knowledge about race and racism is a personal choice that many knowingly make (Mueller, 2020, DeRosa, 2017).

Historical legislative context

Scenario: Abena

You are a student on a ward in a rural part of the country and have been assigned to provide supervised care for Abena, a 25-year-old Black patient who was newly admitted. Your supervisor has asked you to gain information from her to complete the admissions forms. After introducing yourself, to make light conversation, you ask Abena how long she has been studying at the local university and which country she was from. She tells you that she is not a student. She was born in this hospital and still lives with her family in the area. You express your surprise and tell her that most people like her in the neighbourhood are usually students at the university.

Activity 4.1   Decision-making

How else could the above scenario be handled to remove assumptive questions based on a patient presenting as a young Black female?

There is an outline answer to these questions at the end of the chapter.

The presence of people now racialised as minority ethnic in the UK has a long history dating back to Tudor times, which is not always understood or recognised in some instances because it is not taught as part of standard British history in schools (Akala, 2019). However, it is now generally understood that we live in a multicultural society with identifiable and non-identifiable differences among a wide variety of groups in our social system. This diversity has a historical base with Britain as empire, with continued links that were responsible for eventually creating a 'Commonwealth of Nations', overseen by the British monarchy as head of state. Consequently, Britain regularly called on the people of these nations for post-war support in order to rebuild the UK nations. Acknowledgement of this background is important to ensure that there is clear understanding of the historical context. This also helps to clarify the discourse with respect to refugees and asylum seekers, who are usually escaping war and persecution in their own countries. It is hence expected that every effort is made, especially by those who work in public sector services such as the NHS, to understand how being seen to be different, also referred to as othering, may impact on the lives of individuals and groups in our society. Those who deliver care in the NHS are duty bound by the Nursing and Midwifery Council (NMC, 2023) to ensure that the care they deliver recognises diversity and individual choice, and is free from assumptions about patients, based on how they may present physically, including their race and ethnicity.

The Race Relations Act of 1965 was the first initial driver for change in relation to anti-discriminatory practice across UK society and became necessary because of an increase in race-related incidences that negatively affected Black and Brown communities in the UK. The Act acknowledged that discrimination against these communities had become commonplace across social and institutional structures, and it was made unlawful. This was necessary because large numbers of people from Black and Brown communities around the world, specifically from Africa and the Caribbean, who had settled in the UK, had begun to report discrimination in the workplace. It was followed by the Sex Discrimination Act of 1975. Race hence became one of the protected characteristics of the UK Equality Act (2010), along with gender, disability, religion, and so on, given the continued issues with racial tensions and discrimination in society and in workplaces such as the NHS. It must be emphasised that race as a concept has been challenged and questioned by many scholars as misrepresenting the realities of human behaviours, intelligence and similarities. However, as discussed above, the UK's Race Relations Act of 1965 identified that people groups were the victims of discrimination due to their race, which made it a protected characteristic in the current legislative framework. Ethnicity and ethnic representation tend to be linked to social groupings sharing geographical, linguistic, religious, or historical traditions, which make them different from other groups of people.

What makes people different?

Case study: Jan (Yanique)

Jan (Yanique), is a transgender patient of mixed racial origins who was assigned male at birth. They were admitted to the female surgical ward from the A&E Department for overnight observations. They had suffered only minor injuries from a road traffic accident, however, the doctors wanted to be sure before sending them back home. Jan was placed in a bed on the open ward, alongside two female patients, one on either side.

On arrival you were asked by your supervisor to settle them into bed and take the first observations.

Mrs Lillian Greene, one of the female patients in the bed next to Jan, overheard your conversation with Jan while you performed their assessment and observations. Thinking that Jan is a Black male, she complained that she wished to be moved from that bed as she did not feel safe beside Jan. The woman on the other side of Jan also complained about the 'male' patient on the female ward and requested to be moved.

As a consequence, the decision was made to transfer them to another ward as it was not felt that the current environment was suitable for them.

Activity 4.2   Reflection

Share your thoughts about transgender patients' presence on wards classified for male or female patients. Should it matter? Discuss this with your peers, supervisor and tutor.

Think about how else this scenario might have been managed on the ward.

As this activity is based on your own reflection, there is no outline answer.

Difference as a concept and lived reality for many people may manifest itself in a variety of ways in society. For example, people from various parts of Europe who present as White, may identify differently when they speak or by their name. It is now acknowledged that individual accents can have a negative impact on how people are perceived and understood. It is also known that society favours some accents above others, which makes it possible to treat people differently because of the way they speak (Brown 2022, Sharma et al., 2022). People from parts of Asia may be identifiable by the way they dress, their speech and their skin colour, in some cases. The same is true of some refugees who arrive from different parts of the world. Second and third generation people from Europe likely speak with local British accents that do not identify them as different. But people who are originally from Africa and the Caribbean, many of whom are also second and third generation, are often immediately visibly identifiable as being Black or Brown. They are usually fluent in English; however, this does not diminish the negative impact on their experiences in society. According to most of the current research Black and Brown people are noted as having differential discriminatory outcomes across the social structure, including in healthcare (Thompson, 2021). What this identifies is that there are other underlying factors that influence the way they are perceived as individuals or as part of a group. Being racialised as Black or Brown therefore carries negative connotations that affect their whole life experiences, whether this is in education, health, or social care.

The Equality Act (2010) is in itself an acknowledgement that we live in a discriminatory society. Legislative protected characteristics aim to ensure that individuals and groups can seek redress legally if they have been harmed by discriminatory actions of others or of institutions such as healthcare. The NHS is identified as one of the biggest employers of minority ethnic people. Being able to also communicate with people from this group effectively as colleagues, has the potential to improve relationships in the workplace and contribute to patient safety (Watson, 2019).

The Covid-19 pandemic affected healthcare systems worldwide and shone a very sharp spotlight on a range of inequitable health outcomes specifically affecting minority ethnic people in the UK's NHS. Mortality rates were reported to be disproportionately higher than in the White population, exposing another sombre statistic of racial health inequalities (Raleigh and Holmes, 2021).

Given the continuous challenges of poor and inequitable outcomes for minority ethnic users of healthcare services (NHS England and Improvement NHS, 2020; Department of Health and Social Care, 2011), and the events of the recent pandemic and the BLM movement, a focus on race and its impact on interethnic communication in this chapter is aimed at providing a context that can facilitate further thinking, reflection and action for students and staff.

In addition to the points raised above, the case study below aims to put this into context.

Case study: Sickle cell anaemia: Steven Nathan Smith's dilemma

In 2019, Steven Nathan Smith, a young British-born Black student in his twenties, was admitted to an NHS hospital suffering from a sickle cell crisis. He was treated initially and was then observed as an inpatient. While in hospital, he became very distressed and went into a further sickling crisis.

He was unable to breathe and needed oxygen urgently. He called for help, but no one responded. In a state of desperation, he dialled 999 from his hospital bed. He eventually died before he was given any assistance (Sickle Cell Society, 2021). He was British-born and raised, yet he was ignored by staff when he called out for help as he struggled to breathe.

This incident raises many questions that all staff must reflect on and address in order to ensure that such an incident will not happen again.

But what are the lessons that may be learnt and how might they be addressed?

Activity 4.3   Communication

1. What should be an appropriate response by staff when any patient rings a bell or calls out for help on a hospital ward?
2. Thinking about the above scenario, consider the likely reasons why Steven was ignored when he cried out for help. Are they justifiable?
3. When you get some time, read the full report on this tragic case to gain further insights into how this could have been better managed. The report details can be found in the Further reading section of this chapter.

There is an outline answer to these questions at the end of the chapter.

Sickle cell disease is common among African and Caribbean people, and those from Mediterranean backgrounds. Approximately 17,500 people live with the disorder in the UK and around 300 babies are born with the disease annually. The illness is characterised by a sickling of the red blood cells which reduces their oxygen-carrying capacity and can then cause blockages in the circulatory system. The reduced oxygen can be detrimental to breathing and patients need oxygen therapy as a matter of urgency. There is also usually intense pain as clumped cells struggle to move around the body, making patients very distressed. Along with sickle cell disease, other illnesses that are common among minority ethnic communities include thalassaemia, hypertension and type 2 diabetes (Raleigh and Holmes, 2021).

As a student, it is important to make opportunities to learn about the way that these diseases affect minority ethnic communities. The aim is to improve and build on clinical skills while learning about the best ways to communicate with patients. This includes some measure of self-awareness in order to recognise what barriers may be interfering with your ability to not only listen to all patients, but to hear and respond to them.

Stockwell (1972) was one of the very first nurse researchers to identify that nurses classify patients as popular or unpopular based on certain features such as being easy to get on with, being helpful on wards or not complaining even if they should. They were then treated favourably or not, depending on how nurses perceived them. Unpopular patients were ignored in some cases. Ethnicity was also cited in the Black Report (1980) which identified minority ethnic patients as having differential outcomes as a result of unequal care in the NHS. These research papers provided early signposts to the issues that contribute to health inequalities. It is interesting that in the twenty-first century, the problem of unequal access persists, and indeed, appears to be getting worse. It is up to everyone to consider what preconceived assumptions may be interfering with their ability to hear and listen to the voices of minority ethnic patients. This issue is particularly worrying considering there are also migrant communities who may be trying to be understood through a potential language barrier. There is an established Black British community in the UK who have no difficulty with the use of English as a language and are still not being heard. The enquiry into Steven's death concluded that the delivery of care was substandard and failed to meet his health needs.

Cultural competence and care delivery

This is defined as being able to effectively respond to the needs of people from a variety of backgrounds and cultures so that the care provided and services being delivered adequately meet both communication and cultural needs (Papadopolous, 2011).

Cultural competence enables nurses and healthcare workers to become more efficient and empathetic when providing care to patients from diverse backgrounds, especially related to their racial differences. To enable this, nurses need to understand and appreciate the differences in terms of health beliefs and practices that are likely to affect interethnic communication style. Some time must be spent learning about ethnic differences in health and disease processes in order to deliver effective care. Nurses also need to understand the impact of racialisation on minority ethnic patients and how this may affect their access to care and services. Showing awareness will contribute to helping to ensure that the care being delivered is not only fair and equitable but is also effective and suitable for the needs of the patient. To enable this process, interethnic communication must include the decision to make sure that the patient's needs can be understood from their perspectives. Care can then be delivered without bias or assumptions. To do this effectively involves an awareness of one's own personal and cultural values and beliefs, including ways that these may differ from other cultures. It also acknowledges that the dominant culture in the care context may not always reflect the needs of those who are culturally different without intentional actions on the part of nurses. Within nursing and healthcare practice, this awareness enables staff to provide good quality care to patients by demonstrating clear understanding of issues such as likely differences in health beliefs and practices including having a knowledge base about other people's cultural practices and the way they think. Additionally, it helps us to modify our attitudes towards cultural differences and make us more willing to understand and respect diverse relationships. Developing cross cultural, or intercultural skills from a knowledge base has the potential to contribute to improved clinical practice, patient satisfaction and quality of care.

Scenario: Kofi's cardiac arrest

Kofi is a patient with a dark skin tone, who was admitted to your ward having suffered a mild heart attack. He has stabilised over a 24-hour period but is being kept in for further observations and medical checks prior to being discharged the next day. He rings his bell and when you respond he complains of shortness of breath and says he is unable to breathe. However, when you look at him you are not sure because he looks exactly the same as he has since admission. You inform your supervisor who says Kofi is doing well and will be going home the next day. When you return to his bedside you notice that he appears to be asleep, but on further checking, he has collapsed and stopped breathing.

Activity 4.4   Decision-making

1. What signs should you look for to help you identify what is wrong with this patient?
2. How will you attempt to verify what he says?
3. Why is this important for a patient whose skin tone is dark?

An outline answer is given at the end of the chapter.

It has long been argued that skills-based competencies are reflective of the majority of the population and do not adequately cater for minority ethnic people in the community. Biases based on racial disparities are well documented in all aspects of healthcare. This includes pain assessment and management, and access to surgical procedures and medications (Nyguyen et al., 2023). For example, a White patient who lacks oxygen will look pale and blue. But it is not always clear if nurses are aware of how a patient with a darker skin tone may present if their oxygen levels are low.

Unconscious bias

Whether or not we are aware, our style of communication is heavily driven by a number of behaviours and attitudes which may be transmitted to patients and colleagues either positively or negatively. They may originate from our past-life experiences, our personal preferences, our personal beliefs and values, covert, or overt messages we have been given from social or family environments and the stereotypes that we have built up as a result. Unconscious bias is a term which is used to identify behaviours that may be caused by subconscious messages we receive from others and from our environment and upbringing, based on the areas just outlined. These messages drive the way an individual responds to others and have the potential of negatively disadvantaging them as a result. In the context of understanding bias, however, authors such as (Borschman and Marino, 2019) argue that using the term unconscious bias is simply a distraction that unfairly releases some people from taking responsibility for deliberate discriminatory actions to any of the protected characteristics identified by the Equality Act (2010) and including sexual orientation. As discussed in Chapter 1, developing and strengthening your self-awareness is one way of addressing your personal contribution to how your communication is interpreted by others. This is vital when working within the healthcare context.

Why it is important and how it is manifested

Caring for all patients requires an understanding of sociocultural factors that may have an impact on many aspects of their lives. In the case of patients who are visible minorities, meaning that they are immediately identifiable as Black or Brown and hence seen as other, there is a risk of possible unconscious bias, which could be manifested in the way they are treated. Research suggests that social racialisation processes that label visible minorities as drug addicts, underachievers and troublemakers. This labelling is likely to influence the way visible minorities are perceived across institutions and this is likely to have a major negative impact on how they are treated when they attempt to access nursing, health, social care and other services (Thompson, 2021).

Understanding the likely impact on patient experience has the potential to contribute to better nursing care outcomes in all healthcare contexts. Consider the scenario below as an example.

Scenario: Patricia's pain

It is your first day on the medical ward and you are accompanying your supervisor who is conducting the medication round. Patricia, a 21-year-old African Caribbean woman, who lives with systemic lupus erythematosus (SLE) was admitted that morning.

SLE is a debilitating illness which is very common among people of African and Caribbean origins. It manifests itself in intensely painful and swollen joints, muscular pain, body rashes and extreme persistent tiredness. It also causes chest pains and may lead to damage to the kidneys.

Patricia was admitted because of a flare-up of the condition. She presented with excessively swollen joints and was unable to walk because of the pain. She was running a high fever and had some skin lesions on her face and arms. She complained of chest pains and being unable to urinate. She had been immediately catheterised on admission to relieve her bladder distension and was being strictly monitored from a fluid balance perspective, on account of her chest pains, and the possibility of pleurisy, or excessive fluid on the lungs.

She has been on the ward for four hours and asks for pain relief for very panful joints. Your supervisor looks at her prescription chart and notices that her last medication for pain relief was two hours previously. It is prescribed to be given whenever necessary. Your supervisor advises Patricia that she should wait for a while longer as the drug she has been prescribed is very addictive and she may become dependent on it. Patricia says she is in a lot of pain and needs help now. Your supervisor responds that she doesn't look like she is in pain and carries on with the medication round.

Activity 4.5   Decision-making

What can you, as a student nurse, do for this patient?

There is an outline answer to this question at the end of the chapter.

Unconscious bias in care delivery practice must be recognised and acted on by those who deliver care to diverse patients. It may be necessary to undertake training to raise awareness that can positively influence a change in care delivery practice to make sure that minority ethnic patients who present with pain are listened to and can receive pain relief when they request it. To assume that they may be previous drug users or have become addicted due to overmedication is to cause harm to the patient by prolonging their agony. This has the potential to have a very negative impact on patient satisfaction. Unconscious bias may also interfere with your communication with your colleagues who are from different cultures, or even from a different part of the UK, therefore it is important to consider what kinds of bias may be manifested about people from the North, as opposed to those from the South. Issues relating to the inequity in healthcare related to a North/South divide is well documented.

Intersectionality, social justice and antiracist practice

Intersectionality is a term used to identify the likely effects of one or more factors that may be experienced in a discriminatory way by individuals. The term originated in America and was initially used to describe the impact of multiple oppressive actions on Black women's experiences (Crenshaw, 1989, Merz et al., 2023). It is now widely discussed and accepted as an important issue to be considered when exploring oppressive actions on lived experiences of those who have multiple diverse backgrounds. For example, the impact of gender, race and social class each brings with them specific varied responses that are likely to cause harm to the individual patient. A minority ethnic female patient who is also gay, transgender and disabled is likely to feel the oppressive effects of all four characteristics that intersect. This is particularly relevant in relation to access to services and has to be considered when caring for such patients. The same is true for an older minority ethnic female patient. It is likely that conscious or unconscious bias may also influence how the patient is perceived and could impact on how she experiences care. An awareness of these issues should enable a better understanding of inclusive ways to care for such patients.

Case study: Jonathan's experience

Jonathan is a Black patient, who is also gay and autistic, and who was admitted to the ward for investigations. His partner wanted to stay with him while he was an inpatient, however, this was not allowed. Jonathan became very difficult and uncooperative, and the staff branded him a troublemaker and called the police following an incident on the ward. No one called Jonathan's partner, who could have helped to reduce the tension.

Activity 4.6   Team working

Outline how this case could have been managed to have a more positive outcome.

There is an outline answer to this question at the end of the chapter.

Addressing communication issues to improve interethnic care delivery practices

As a student nurse, you will have many learning opportunities to practise your communication skills, in practice and in your learning environment. This book provides the theoretical base for you to further explore and build on your skills. To improve your understanding, you will be required to be ready and willing to face up to sometimes difficult issues that are clearly evidenced in the research and literature base. Health inequalities are well documented, and as it is now an accepted fact that our social and institutional structures tend to be discriminatory, it is then up to us to take action to change the narrative. One way of doing this is to begin by owning up to your own individual biases and tendencies to treat others differently. You may be showing unconscious bias. However, this is something you can act on and the next scenario is a helpful example of what you can do.

Scenario: Sam's peer-to-peer discussion

You are with a group of your student peers; your tutor is not present. Sam, who is in the group and is from London, started a discussion about personal biases by saying that she cannot cope with Northerners because she just cannot understand them when they speak. She also said she struggles with refugees and people with deep accents, and that she found it difficult to understand a couple of the foreign doctors on the ward. You are surprised by this and ask her to explain. She said she had been reading up about biases and thought she should own up to some that she has.

Activity 4.7   Reflection

- Share some of your biases with your peers if you can. Only share what you are comfortable with.

- Consider where Sam may have got her biases from, or what may have contributed to them.

- Talk to the group about other ways that you can all address your biases, especially at work.

As this activity is based on your own observation, there is no outline answer.

Chapter summary

Most minority ethnic patients are able to eventually gain access to health and care services when they present during their illness. However, there is now overwhelming evidence that the way they are treated during the care delivery process is causing harm to their wellbeing, leading to increased mortality. This needs to immediately improve across all sectors of the health and care systems (Thompson, 2021).

Listening to and hearing the voices of minority ethnic people who try to access health and social care, or other services, is imperative if the goal of healthcare is to ensure equity and accountability (NHS England and NHS Improvement, 2021a). Any reluctance or resistance from health service staff can be a matter of life and death, as illustrated in some cases discussed in this chapter. There are still major barriers that negatively impact care quality outcomes for Black patients. This may be conscious or unconscious bias, intersectionality, racialisation and racism which leads to unequal outcomes in their experiences and undermines the quality of expected care. It is up to each individual practitioner to ensure that there is awareness of the current evidence which is now widely available relating to inequalities in access and healthcare delivery. Nursing and healthcare workers are required to strive to be a part of the solution by changing the narrative and ensuring best practice is maintained at all times. One way of doing this is to hold each individual accountable and also to monitor, measure and penalise, if necessary, all negative outcomes for all patients. Facing up to the evidence and taking action to mitigate the continuous negative impact of race, racism and racialisation in healthcare services is the duty of everyone, including you as a student, your supervisor in clinical practice and the institution. Becoming a diversity champion in your unit is another proactive way of contributing to the solution in the workplace.

Activities: brief outline answers

Activity 4.1 (page 53)

You are likely to meet minority ethnic patients in many settings, rural or urban. Never assume that they are foreigners by asking leading questions, except where required for assessment purposes.

Activity 4.3 (page 56)

You will know that every patient who rings a bell or calls for help should be given an immediate response. This can be crucial to life or death, and until someone has attended the patient and assessed the situation it is not possible to know what state they may be in. There are no justifiable reasons to ignore any patient's call when they ring a ward bell.

Activity 4.4 (page 58)

As this is a patient with a dark skin tone, you should expect his face to look grey.

You should check his oxygen levels with an oximeter, as a standard aspect of care.

This is important because you will likely be familiar with caring for patients with White skins and may not be aware of how the facial skin of a darker skin-toned patient may change if they are oxygen starved. A White patient's skin may turn blue/pale when oxygen starved.

You should also immediately talk to your supervisor about the patient's complaint and ensure that someone senior checks that your observations are correct and appropriate.

For this patient this could be a matter of life and death and should not be taken lightly, especially given the well-known evidence that Black patients have differential and inequitable outcomes in care delivery practice.

Activity 4.5 (page 60)

The patient has had a two-hour gap since the last medication was given. It is prescribed to be given whenever necessary. Your supervisor should therefore respond by giving the patient her medication as prescribed.

Understanding the impact of SLE on all patients, but specifically on African Caribbean patients, who are most likely to present, is important when caring for those who live with this condition. The evidence identifies that healthcare professionals have a tendency not to believe these patients when they say they are in pain.

As a student, you can make some time to find out more about the illness if you have not yet done this in your studies. If you have covered the topic, you may be able to discuss this with your supervisor and be an advocate for the patient. Being an advocate simply means speaking on behalf of the patient, a role that you may already have practised with other patients. This need not be difficult or challenging and could simply be a matter of informing your supervisor that in your studies you had read about this condition and how important it was to ensure that all patients receive pain relief when they ask for it. You could offer to speak about the illness at the next staff meeting and prepare a teaching pack for ward staff. You could contact the SLE society and arrange for them to deliver a training session to the staff. This proactive action could form part of a case study for your studies, as long as you ensure that your supervisor and the patient give permission, and confidentiality is maintained.

Activity 4.6   (page 61)

Working towards positive outcomes in healthcare delivery requires sensitivity in the way all patients are treated. Since this patient had been declared as having an autistic spectrum disorder, is Black, and has a same sex partner, there may be issues of inequity creeping in that staff should be aware of. For example, it is unclear why they would wish to deny his partner access when he could be a supportive presence that could allay the patient's fears and reduce his anxiety. Hospitals are stressful environments for most patients, especially those who are neurodivergent. To be Black and gay also brings with it multiple discriminatory perspectives that staff should be aware of and seek to mitigate. To call security and not to call his partner is inexplicable and unnecessary.

Further reading

Allen, H and Taylor, M (eds) (2023) *Researching Racism in the NHS: Reflexive Accounts and Personal Stories.* London: Taylor & Francis.

This test explores the impact of racism and microaggressions in the NHS, on individual experiences.

Kinouani, G (2021) *Living While Black: The Essential Guide to Overcoming Racial Trauma.* London: Penguin Random House.

Covers experiences of Black people and ways that they adapt to overcome daily racialised life events.

Llewelyn, S and Packer, S (2021) *Still Breathing: 100 Black Voices on Racism, 100 Ways to Change the Narrative.* London: Harper Collins.

Considers the experiences of prominent Black voices and how they overcome racialisation.

Sickle Cell Society (2021) No One's Listening - A Report. Available at: www.sicklecellsociety.org/no-ones-listening/ (Accessed 15 January 2024).

Weir, MR (2020) *I Can't Breathe. Can 8 Minutes 46 Seconds Change the World?* London: Krik Krak.

Uses artistic imagery to highlight race implications following George Floyd's death.

The full report providing detailed context and findings of the report into the death of Steven, a young Black man, while in hospital from a sickle cell crisis.

Useful websites

www.open.ac.uk/black-womens-health-and-wellbeing

Black women's health and wellbeing research network. A knowledge hub on developments, resources and evidence on Black women's health in the UK, North, South, Middle America and the Caribbean.

www.npeu.ox.ac.uk/mbrrace-uk/reports

MBRRACE-UK – saving lives, improving mothers' care. Report on Black maternal mortality in the UK.

www.sicklecellsociety.org/

Sickle Cell Society (2021) Supporting the Black community. Providing helpful information about this disease for sufferers, carers and members of the public.

Chapter 5

Communication and the multidisciplinary team

Paulette Johnson

Chapter aims

....

After reading this chapter, you will be able to:

- define what a multidisciplinary (MDT) team is;
- understand the possible range of professionals involved in an MDT;
- understand the functions of an MDT;
- learn more about the issues that influence communication within the MDT;
- appreciate the importance of engagement with family and carers when working within an MDT;
- consider leadership and management in overseeing MDTs.

Introduction

Life often involves complexity; any one individual may have more than one need or issue requiring support or intervention. If we are to think about how we can best support an individual in a holistic way, considering all areas of someone's life and having consideration of how one element of life impacts another, it is important that we think about the whole person, typically described as a *holistic* way of working. If we fail to consider all needs the likelihood is that that person will not be able to make a full recovery, or even function to their full potential in society. For these reasons, it's important to come together as a group of professionals to support an individual with their range of needs. In the field of health and social care working jointly as a group of professionals is referred to as working as a multidisciplinary team (MDT). Multidisciplinary team (MDT) is the generic term used to describe teams of professionals with different expertise that are set up to collectively coordinate and deliver health and care services for individuals, particularly in circumstances where an individual has complex health and care needs. Across the UK each of the countries approach elements of their health and care systems in this way. Each of the countries have made a commitment to work together with other professionals to provide integrated care and support to those patients who have complex and multiple needs, which we will explore this later in the chapter. In terms of good practice guidance, the Social Care Institute for Excellence (SCIE) provides health and social care professionals across the UK with guidance on how we can best work to support the communities we serve. MDTs are endorsed by SCIE as an approach to working that provides improved health and wellbeing for individuals, enhanced care, good value, good quality and sustainable care (SCIE, 2022a).

As a student nurse, you may question why working in this way is necessary and why one professional is not able to support an individual with the range of needs they may present with. This chapter explores the functions of the MDT and the possible roles that make up a team of professionals using this approach to working within different contexts, providing a basis for why this approach to working provides positive outcomes for the people we are working with. Communication and information sharing are key aspects of the MDT approach, which this chapter will explore in detail as well as how the process of joint working is managed effectively. Service users and their loved ones are key to the joint working relationship so we will also look at best practice approaches to working in this way. In conclusion we look at the universal approach to MDTs and the legislative frameworks across the UK touching on innovation in this area of work.

Below is a case study that will help you start to think about the complex needs you may be presented with in practice.

Case study: Tinashe

Tinashe attended the endocrinology clinic where he has an appointment with the specialist nurse team. Tinashe's main issue is his thyroid function and many of the resulting health issues are associated with noncompliance of the daily medication regime required to maintain his health. Tinashe also has a severe learning disability so is supported by his mother who is his main carer. Ola (Tinashe's mum) has explained to health professionals that it has become increasingly difficult to encourage Tinashe to take his medication daily as he has got older and his understanding of the impact this is having on his health is limited. Tinashe is now morbidly obese; he suffers with severe muscle aching which is affecting his mobility significantly and he is very tired most of the time, which is now limiting his social interaction. The endocrinology clinic will continue to work with Tinashe but a holistic approach to managing his care may be more beneficial to his health.

Activity 5.1   Critical thinking

Thinking about the pros (positives) and cons (limitations) of working one-to-one with Tinashe, or as part of a wider team: Consider the following questions and discuss them with your supervisor or a fellow student.

- What are the pros of working with Tinashe one-to-one in the endocrinology clinic? What are the cons?
- What are the pros of working with a team of professionals to support Tinashe? What are the cons?
- How might these pros be achieved?

There is an outline answer to these questions at the end of the chapter.

Understanding the possible range of professionals involved in the MDT

You should now understand the benefits of working together as professionals so we are going to go on to look at which professionals might be involved in working together.

Activity 5.2   Reflection

Thinking about the case study involving Tinashe above.

- Can you list the professionals that might need to be involved in working with Tinashe to ensure all his needs are met?

There is usually a lead person who acts as the principal or lead case manager when professionals are working in an MDT. Who becomes the lead person for care may depend on the needs of the individual being cared for. If an individual has significant healthcare needs, the MDT may be led by healthcare professionals involved with care. If the needs of the individual being cared for are more related to social care, you may find that social care professionals are the lead case managers. If there is a legal requirement for engagement with services (an example of this may be safeguarding or criminal justice interventions) these professionals may take on the role of principal case manager.

The principal case manager has a key role in leading the MDT.

- What responsibilities do you think are key to the role of principal or lead case manager?

There is an outline answer to these questions at the end of the chapter.

You have now learned that MDTs consist of professionals across different disciplines and can include professionals employed in public services and private and voluntary sector agencies. Later in the chapter we will look at case examples of multidisciplinary teams and explore the roles some of these professionals undertake in working towards a common goal of supporting an individual.

The size and composition of the MDT can vary depending on service and locality. Within a commissioning area there are usually teams that are already working collaboratively, however, where there is a need to engage an additional specialist service this can be agreed amongst the team. Whether a service can work with the MDT will depend on their agreement with funders of the service they provide. If the team has capacity to get involved, their geographical location and whether the individual in need meets that threshold as set out in the service specification are all contributing factors. The service specification threshold does sometimes mean that some individuals are deemed ineligible for a particular service, but it remains the responsibility of the MDT to explore suitable alternatives.

A conversation with your supervisor

Your clinical supervisor or an experienced nurse colleague will have experience of being part of an MDT. Here you will get an opportunity to talk to them directly about this and learn more about how an MDT works in a practice setting.

Activity 5.3   Team working

Arrange time at your next supervision meeting or with a colleague. Explain that you are learning more about working in an MDT and that you would like to talk with them about their experience of working in this way.

Suggestion for your agenda:

- How long have you been a professional nurse?
- Have you been part of an MDT in your role as a nurse? If not, how have you worked collaboratively with colleagues to support an individual?
- What are the benefits of working in an MDT/or working collaboratively?
- Are there any limitations in working as part of an MDT, or working collaboratively to support an individual?

Come back to your group and have a discussion with your peers about the conversations you have had with nursing colleagues.

1. Did you identify any benefits to working in an MDT?
2. Did you identify any limitations to working in an MDT?

You will see some examples of the kind of information you might gather at the end of the chapter.

Issues that influence communication within the MDT

You may well have discussed issues of communication when you were thinking about the limitations and benefits of working in an MDT. Effective communication is key to delivering high-quality care and to ensuring delivery of safe and effective care. When we talked about the functions of the MDT you will have noticed that there are elements of that work that required clear and effective communication within the team and with external people or agencies involved in the care and treatment of the person at the centre of the care plan. NHS England provide guidance for service users and for healthcare workers (NHS England and NHS Improvement, 2019). This outlines what the legal responsibilities of healthcare providers are as far as managing and storing information relating to the person being cared for. Healthcare professionals must only share information that is necessary, and any such information should be relevant to the work being undertaken. This guidance is compliant with the UK General Data Protection Regulation and the Data Protection Act 2018 that provides a legal framework for keeping personal information safe and outlines processes for handling and storing personal information. In a hospital setting or a large organisation, professionals can seek advice about information sharing from a Caldicott Guardian of the organisation. In small organisations or non-hospital settings there will be a designated person who deals with information governance. Most organisations require all staff to compete General Data Protection Regulation (GDPR) training as part of any induction and mandatory training and this should be updated periodically. This ensures that professionals are clear about how they should manage personal information and colleagues specialising in this work can be a useful point of contact if you are in doubt about who to share information with, how long to store information and what to do in the event of a possible breach of information.

Understanding the functions of the MDT

Ultimately the MDT exists to support the health and care of an individual in a coordinated way to achieve the best outcomes, however, in order to achieve that, the MDT has several functions. In some cases, these include specific tasks, but other functions may take the form of a process that will need to be formalised and clear for all parties involved.

The functions of the MDT fit under the following broad areas:

- liaison and advice;
- clinical;
- interventions;
- referral;
- data collection and monitoring;
- safeguarding.

Tasks and functions of the MDT

The make-up of the MDT allows for optimisation of coordinated care that is responsive to an individual's needs, very much aligned to person-centred approaches to care (Rogers, 1951). Here are further details about each of the above roles:

1. Liaison and advice functions

    This function specifically relates to information, advice and guidance. Central to the process is the individual in need of care but there is also the family and/or carer to consider: it is crucial that these individuals are valued as part of the process and are included in decision-making with the consent of the individual being cared for. Ensuring allied professionals and private and voluntary sector organisations are included in the process and are able to share their expertise is of high importance. Liaison outside of the MDT may include services such as housing, education, legal services, etc. where there is no representation within the MDT.

2. Clinical functions

This can include screening, triage, medical intervention, psycho-social assessment or facilitating specialist assessment for intervention as appropriate and/or needed.

3. Intervention functions

As there are specialist and professionally qualified members of the MDTs it may be the case that the short-term interventions are delivered by members within the team. This allows for direct reporting to the MDT and provides first-hand experience of working directly with an individual. This can produce accurate and in-depth feedback which is very useful to the MDT.

4. Referral functions

When making referrals, there is a need to identify and agree different pathways for an individual's care. Members of the MDT facilitate referrals and follow these up within and outside of the MDT. It is important to ensure specialist services and support is engaged where necessary to achieve more detailed assessment, particularly in relation to highly complex needs. Collation of information on outcomes (to and from the referring agency) requires the necessary information sharing protocols and individual consent, allowing professionals to share information for specific purposes.

5. Data collection and monitoring functions

This can involve tracking the progress of the individual being supported to assess the impact and effectiveness of the interventions/support being offered and delivered. Additionally, monitoring of equal opportunities information can promote inclusion and identify any patterns or trends that can be acted on to promote equality and diversity. Case management and data reporting are also important to evidence service delivery outcomes according to the service requirements agreed with commissioners.

6. Safeguarding functions

It is important to ensure that service policies and procedures are followed appropriately and that any concerns relating to safeguarding are appropriately reported and/or acted on.

7. Remit and time frames

The MDT can provide care and support for individuals within the hospital setting, but this care and support can also be in place following hospital discharge and whilst the individual being cared for is in the community. The time frame that an MDT works with an individual can be informed by patient need and agreed with the team. In some cases, services have specific time frames within which they can provide care and support.

In order to be an effective MDT and provide a good level of service to those in need of care, it should have processes that make provision for effective meetings. As with any meeting, there should be a clear purpose, agreed aims and specific objectives.

Activity 5.4   Reflection

Think about a time when you were part of a meeting, whether in a hospital setting or in another care setting.

Identify the actions that made this meeting effective.

There is an outline answer to these questions at the end of the chapter.

The planning and organisation of the meeting is as important as how the meeting is managed and what outcomes are agreed. It is important to think about the experience of the person being cared for and to ensure the MDT is clear that the needs of those being cared for are met. The meeting is the record of planning and decision-making and is the forum within which agreed actions are measured and evaluated. As well as recording minutes of the meeting, this is usually the place to complete a care plan for the person being cared for. In formulating a care plan the MDT will agree a set of objectives; these will form goals to work towards in the short term and longer term. In setting goals, it is good practice to follow a set of principles known as SMART objectives (Doran, 1981).

The acronym outlines the following principles:

Specific: the objectives should state what it is that is aiming to be achieved;

Measurable: the objective should have a measure that indicates how the MDT will know that the objective has been met;

Achievable: it must be possible to achieve the objective within the plan set out by the MDT and resources needed to achieve the objective should be clear;

Realistic: the objective should be realistic for the person being cared for and the remit and responsibilities of the MDT;

Timebound: the time frame for the objective should be clearly stated. This could be short term. This could be at a fixed point in the long term or the short term.

(Adapted from Doran, G.T., 1981)

Below is a case study which will help you to explore how an MDT could support an individual who presents with varied and complex needs. You can approach this exercise on your own or in a group.

Case study: George

George is 65 years old and has been maintained on methadone for several years. He is single but has a son (Tom) who is registered as George's main carer. George developed a back condition when he worked in the mines and never recovered.

George's condition has been maintained with medication for several years and George has gone through periods where he has used illegal drugs, in an attempt to manage the pain. This has resulted in him injecting drugs, which has led to him developing deep vein thrombosis and he now risks leg amputation.

George's general health is deteriorating, and he has been admitted to hospital for treatment.

He lives in social housing and is in receipt of state benefits. He has been in hospital longer than the period for which state benefits can be paid to an individual.

Activity 5.5   Decision-making

- Which services do you think would form part of a team suitably qualified and experienced to coordinate care for George?
- Which external agencies might the MDT need to liaise with?
- In what way would the MDT involve George's carer (Tom)? Would there be any considerations?

There is an outline answer to these questions at the end of the chapter.

Although George's drug use and the problems he is now experiencing as a result are closely connected with his healthcare needs, there are specialist drug and alcohol professionals who can best provide advice and guidance on harm minimisation (a preventative approach to working with drug misusers) to prevent any further harm or relapse to previous drug misusing behaviours.

George is at risk of losing his accommodation, so a specialist housing advice worker could support George with his housing options and in working towards finding suitable accommodation.

As George is classed as an adult with additional needs, he will be entitled to an assessment under the Care Act (Legislation.gov.uk, 2014a), and this would be undertaken by a social work professional. This will identify what support the local authority have a duty to provide. Tom (who may or may not be a registered carer) is entitled to a carer's assessment to have his needs assessed and ensure that he is appropriately registered and supported.

As George is in receipt of state benefits, it would be helpful to have an advice worker who can support him with advice about his benefit entitlements whilst in hospital and on return to the community.

George is an inpatient so will also have health professionals working with him, possibly in primary and secondary care services. Once he is well enough for hospital discharge there may also be district nurses involved in his care and rehabilitation.

This is an example of a team of people coming together with different specialisms to support someone with complex needs.

Person-centred/personalised care

The origins of person-centred approaches to working with people came from the seminal work of Carl Rogers (1951). The basis of this approach lies in humanistic philosophy and asserts that given the right conditions, an individual can reach their full potential, referred to in the Rogerian approach as self-actualisation. The principles of this approach are commonly used as the basis for many approaches to counselling and approaches to working with people. They have formed the basis of service design and delivery across the UK and even worldwide. The person-centred approach has many interpretations and how the approach has evolved has no agreed definition as such. This is not surprising given that the fundamental principles of the approach respond to any one individual need, so it would be perfectly reasonable to suggest that person-centred care and what that means would evolve and change over time, as does human life, behaviour and attitudes.

You will have realised now that the MDT approach has a focus on responding to multiple needs of an individual in such a way that allows for these different needs to be responded to by professionals with specific and relevant expertise. This approach is often referred to as person-centred care which is at the heart of the MDT approach to working. The Coalition for Personalised Care (CPC), which is an organisation working closely with NHS England, has set out its shared ambition for personalised care as a universal goal across the health and social care sector. Below is a summary of the vision of what achieving good, personalised care, developed in consultation with service users looks like. The objectives the CPC has developed provide us with an explanation of what personalised care is from the perspective of service users. The CPC have established that most service users want the following as part of personalised care:

- To be treated by professionals they trust as a whole person who has valuable skills, experience and strengths.
- To be able to readily access information and advice that is timely, clear and works for them.
- To be valued as an active participant in all conversations and decisions about their health and wellbeing.

- To be supported to understand their care and support options, and able to set and achieve their personal desired outcomes.
- To be offered a coordinated approach that is transparent and empowering, with their preferences being recorded and remembered.
- To be connected with health coaching, self-management and/or community support programmes.

(Coalition for Personalised Care (n.d.))

You can find more information about person-centred care in the additional resources section of this chapter.

Engagement with family and carers when working

Again, thinking about George's case study, Tom's role as a carer is very important and we are going to think more about how best to facilitate Tom's involvement in the whole process and in decision-making.

The individual being cared for is at the centre of care and support within the MDT but there is also a wider network in the case of many individuals, so involving carers or significant others in the care plan can be extremely beneficial to the individual at the centre of care and is also an important part of the work to support an individual.

Researching carer involvement

Activity 5.6   Evidence-based practice and research

Nicholson, C (2016) How Do We Facilitate Carers' Involvement in Decision-making? *Nursing Older People*, 28(3), pp. 14–14. Available at: doi.org/10.7748/nop.28.3.14.s21.

Read this short article in which the author reflects how we can best facilitate the involvement of family and friends as carers when working with older people via three case studies.

- What observations did the author make in terms of collaboration between relatives of older patients and nurses?
- What methods of carer engagement were found in the care of older people?
- How can nursing professionals best facilitate carers' involvements in decision-making within a hospital setting?

There is an outline answer to these questions at the end of the chapter.

You should now have a grasp of how best we can involve and facilitate carers in the care and decision-making of their loved ones. What should also be apparent is that communication is a key factor in how we achieve this successfully as well as how far we consult with service users. What you have noted is evidence-based good practice guidance, so the principles of this can be used in your work going forward. As we know, things change over time and individuals have different preferences based on several factors. With this in mind, the most suitable approach in most cases is to be led by the needs and wants of the service users you are working with.

Leadership, management and innovation

We have talked at length about the benefits of professionals working together and collectively in MDTs. There are clear benefits for the communities we serve and when delivered well, individuals can have a very positive experience. There is a lot of coordination and planning required when working as an MDT and this happens at different levels of the system. There are Acts (government legislation) and local policies and procedures that provide a framework for and underpin the delivery and development of coordinated care, which we are going to look at in more detail below.

Across the UK governments are moving towards a statutory requirement (legislative requirement) for the health and social care sector to develop integrated care often referred to as welfare reforms. Integrated care is defined by Health Education England (HEE) (2022) as: *care that is planned with people who work together to understand the service user and their carer(s), puts them in control and coordinates and delivers services to achieve the best outcomes.* You will notice that this definition aligns with the approach of MDTs. This follows years of locally led development in the form of MDTs, recommendations from the NHS, consultation with service providers and service users, and evidence of positive outcomes. We are now seeing the development of government legislation that enables local practice that is underpinned by collaborative working between services. Integrated care systems (ICS) is the formal name now given to health and social care organisations in England that are required to come together to form partnerships that plan and deliver care to individuals with care and support needs, again, very much like the approach we see in MDTs. In England we have seen the the Health and Social Care Act (2022) become law on 28 April 2022. This legislation established Integrated Care Boards (ICBs), which abolished CCGs in England (CCGs previously had a role of bringing services together to improve population health and work towards strategic priorities). ICSs have been established across England on a statutory basis from 1 July 2022 (NHS England, 2022) and provide a framework that enables collaborative service delivery at a local level.

There is a UK-wide move towards integrated care:

- In Wales the Social Services and Well-being (Wales) Act 2014 provides for regional partnership boards that bring services together with the purpose of improving outcomes for people with care and support needs.

- In Scotland the Public Bodies (Joint Working) (Scotland) Act 2014 sets out a framework for integrating adult health and social care support.
- In Northern Ireland the Health and Social Care Act 2022 has established ICSs as legal entities.

There is clearly a commitment at the highest level to working in an integrated way, but it is important to recognise that this approach to working requires managers and the front-line professionals involved to embrace this approach and shift the culture from working with individuals on a one-to-one basis (without collaboration) and for organisations to develop systems and processes that support joint working.

Activity 5.7 Critical thinking

- Take a look at the logic model, available at **scie.org.uk** and list at least five benefits of integrated care models.

- If you were in a leadership position, would you prioritise any particular benefits and why?

- Once you have produced a list of at least five benefits of the model, discuss this either in a group or with a partner.

You will be able to identify benefits from the model presented but you may also think of other benefits yourself.

There is an outline answer at the end of the chapter.

In terms of person-centred care or personalised care SCIE (2011) has produced guidance on how professionals might deliver personalised care using a personal budget for each individual, referred to in practice as personalisation. This approach allows service users to take control of their own care and have more flexibility and choice in decisions that are made. Having a personal allocated budget allows service users to make decisions about what support is needed and to be able to think more creatively about their own care. This approach is very innovative in some areas of health and social care and has been trialled across several areas of service delivery, proving to have positive outcomes. You can find more information about this in the useful websites section.

Chapter summary

This chapter has clarified what an MDT is and why this is an approach to working that is being used by health and care professionals across the UK. The activities in this chapter have invited you to explore the benefits and limitations of working in an MDT as well as the different functions of the approach to working, communication across these areas

(Continued)

(Continued)

being a key factor. The chapter has also introduced you to person-centred/personalised best practice approaches to working (Rogers, 1951) that underpin integrated care, as well as practical skills that make for an effective working approach such as SMART objectives (Doran, 1981). There are huge benefits in working in the way that this chapter has touched on and you have also had the opportunity to reflect on the service user perspective and how we can work to better support the populations we serve as health and care professionals. Communication skills will be discussed further in Chapter 8.

Activities: brief outline answers

Activity 5.1   Critical thinking (page 67)

Pros of working with Tinashe one-to-one in the endocrinology clinic	Cons of working one-to-one with Tinashe in the endocrinology clinic
• You can get to know Tinashe and Ola on a one-to-one basis. • Tinashe and Ola feel more comfortable working with the same person. • Tinashe and Ola will not have to repeat more than one assessment. • Tinashe and Ola will have a single point of contact.	• A range of specialist professionals could better understand Tinashe's and Ola's needs. • Tinashe and Ola could benefit from a range of expert support and advice i.e. disability nurse, consultant endocrinologist, social worker/support worker. • Tinashe and Ola can access support from several members of the same team
Pros of working with a team of professionals to support Tinashe	**Cons of working with a team of professionals to support Tinashe**
• Tinashe can benefit from a range of expert advice including: a dietitian, specialist disability nurse, consultant endocrinologist, social worker/support worker. • Different professionals can advocate for Tinashe's different needs and provide specialist advice. • Tinashe and Ola can access support from several members of the same team.	• Tinashe and Ola may be unsure about which professional is working to support them around different issues. • Tinashe and Ola may have concerns about how many times they need to explain and describe their situation. • Members of the MDT might have different goals. • Communication may be complex and will involve the need for information sharing protocols.

Activity 5.2   Reflection (page 68)

1. Professionals who might be involved in Tinashe's care include his GP, an endocrinology nurse, an endocrinology consultant, a dietitian, a social worker, a personal assistant/carer and anoccupational health nurse

2. Any professional member of the team is able to oversee and review the care plan where necessary. Usually the GP or a key worker, if there is one, may be responsible in this case. They are required to communicate with other team members to ensure that the care plan objectives are being met, and will be the main point of contact for Tinashe and Ola.

Activity 5.3   Team working (page 69)

You might find out:

- Which key people need to be involved in the MDT (this could include professionals and any family members or carers).
- Who the MDT will need to agree information sharing protocols with.
- How often the MDT will meet.
- Where the team will meet.
- If there any time frames that the MDT needs to work towards.

Activity 5.4   Reflection (page 72)

- Identify the actions that made this meeting effective.The team are clear about the objectives.
- The objectives are agreed, clear and stated.
- Participants are prepared for the meeting.
- All participants are given an opportunity to participate in a meaningful way.
- The people who need to be involved have been invited to the meeting.
- The meeting is conducted with a clear agenda.
- The meetings start and finish at the agreed time.
- Actions are clear and assigned to individuals.
- All participants are clear about the purpose of the meeting.
- Ensure roles are clearly defined and everyone is clear about the purpose of their contribution.

Activity 5.5   Decision-making (page 73)

- Services forming part of a team suitably qualified to care for George include the GP, the hospital consultant (neurologist, neurosurgeon) specialist nurse, drug worker, benefits advice (citizens advice) social worker.
- External agencies to liaise with include housing, drug and alcohol services, citizens advice, social services. Refer Tom for a carers assessment, Tom can support George with attending appointments, medication compliance, care needs.
- George would need to agree for Tom to be involved in his care.

Activity 5.6   Evidence-based practice and research (page 75)

1. What observations did the author make in terms of collaboration between relatives of older patients and nurses?

    - Carers who collaborated with nurses tended to be more satisfied with their relative's care than those who did not.
    - Low levels of satisfaction were related to low levels of collaboration.
    - Other predictors for low satisfaction were:

        o   feelings of guilt and powerlessness;

        o   helping for less than one year and providing physical care without psycho-social help.

    - Structured involvement of carers is useful in hospital care and during admissions and discharge planning; doing so enables the exchange of information and knowledge and assists in managing expectations.

2. What methods of carer engagement were found in the care of older people?

    - patient caregiving;
    - information sharing;
    - shared decision-making;
    - carer support and education;
    - carer feedback;
    - patient care transitions.

3. How can nursing professionals best facilitate carers' involvements in decision-making within a hospital setting?

- agree procedures or objectives for carer involvement;
- good communication and transparency about how decisions are made;
- management strategies to support nurses and carers to negotiate their involvement openly;
- develop partnerships with carers.

Activity 5.7   Critical thinking (page 77)

- Integrated care improves efficiency by promoting best-value services in the right setting, eliminates service duplication, reduces delays and improves services.
- Effective provision of integrated care helps to manage demand for higher cost hospital care and to control spending growth.
- Integrated care moves resources from higher cost hospital settings to community settings.
- The system enables personalisation by supporting personal budgets.
- It is a cost-effective service model.
- Care is provided in the right place at the right time.
- Demand is well managed.
- It is sustainable care and support.
- You can draw on expertise that you don't have yourself.
- You can access resources that are not available to you in your organisation.
- Resources required to deliver care are shared amongst the stakeholders.

Useful websites

www.england.nhs.uk/publication/making-it-happen-multidisciplinary-team-mdt-working/

Learn more about effective multidisciplinary team working from an English perspective.

www.gov.scot/policies/social-care/

Learn more about social care integration from a Scottish perspective.

www.kingsfund.org.uk/publications/understanding-integration-listen-people-communities

Understanding how to listen to and learn from communities in the development of integrated care systems.

www.nmc.org.uk/standards/code/code-in-action/person-centred-care/

Learn more about person-centred care.

online.hscni.net/our-work/integrated-care-system-ni/

Learn more about integrated care systems in Northern Ireland.

www.personalisedcareinstitute.org.uk/what-is-personalised-care-2/

Learn more about personalised care.

www.scie.org.uk/integrated-care/measuring-evaluating/logic-model

The Social Care Institute for Excellence has developed a tool for organisations to support local planning of integrated care:

www.scie.org.uk/integrated-care/measuring-evaluating/research

Understand more about the government's plans to integrate health and social care.

www.tandfonline.com/doi/abs/10.1080/17571472.2015.11494377

Learn more about integrated care in Wales.

Chapter 6　Communication with children and young people

Liz King

NMC Future Nurse: Standards of Proficiency for Registered Nurses

This chapter will address the following platforms and proficiencies:

Platform 1: Being an accountable professional

1.13　Demonstrate the skills and abilities required to develop, manage and maintain appropriate relationships with people, their families, carers and colleagues.

Platform 2: Promoting health and preventing ill health

2.6　Understand the importance of early years and childhood experiences and the possible impact on life choices, mental, physical and behavioural health and wellbeing.

Platform 3: Assessing needs and planning care

3.16　Demonstrate knowledge of when and how to refer people safely to other professionals or services for clinical intervention or support.

Platform 4: Providing and evaluating care

4.3　Demonstrate the knowledge, communication and relationship management skills required to provide people, families and carers with accurate information that meets their needs before, during and after a range of interventions.

Annexe A: Communication and relationship management skills

2.2　Use clear language and appropriate written materials, making reasonable adjustments where appropriate in order to optimise people's understanding of what has caused their health condition and the implications of their care and treatment.

2.8　Provide information and explanation to people, families and carers and respond to questions about their treatment and care and possible ways of preventing ill health to enhance understanding.

2.9　Engage in difficult conversations, including breaking bad news and support people who are feeling emotionally or physically vulnerable or in distress, conveying compassion and sensitivity.

Chapter aims

After reading this chapter, you will be able to:

- understand why nurses need effective skills for communicating with sick children and young people (CYP) and their families/carers; describe methods of how nurses can communicate compassionately with sick CYP and their families/carers in the acute and community settings reflecting relevant health promotion principles;
- discuss communication aspects relating to safeguarding principles, children in care and the voice of the child;
- identify the importance of multidisciplinary team (MDT) working for communicating with CYP and their families/carers.

Please be aware that the case studies and scenarios detailed in this chapter contain potentially upsetting information for some readers. Please seek support from your university, tutor or supervisor if you are affected by any of the chapter content.

Introduction

The child first and always

(Motto of The Great Ormond Street Hospital for Children)

Case study: Alison

Alison is 14 years old and has been anorexic for five years. Recently, Alison was admitted to her local general children's ward due to being underweight and refusing to eat. The children's nursing team has been caring for Alison with the input of registered mental health nurses and a clinical psychiatrist. There are plans for Alison to be discharged to a special eating disorder unit for further treatment. The bed at the unit is available in three weeks' time and so Alison will remain on the children's ward until then. The nurses will continue to care for Alison, observing her health status and encouraging her to gain an agreed amount of weight. There have been challenges in getting Alison to eat and be weighed daily. In addition, Alison's parents refuse to visit her on the ward, which has upset Alison. At times, Alison has been uncooperative and has attempted to abscond from the ward. Plans for the insertion of a nasogastric tube to feed Alison enterally have now been made as she is not gaining weight sufficiently. The ward-based nurses are not sure if Alison will consent or allow them to pass this tube and the nurses are worried that this action may harm the relationship they have built so far with Alison.

The chapter has started with the above case study, which demonstrates the complexity and importance of communication when nursing children and young people (CYP). Although talking and listening appear to be easy things to do in your everyday life, communication with sick CYP and their families/carers can be challenging, with many factors for nurses to consider. Additionally, nurses have a professional duty to be able to communicate appropriately with their patients and families to ensure that safe and effective care is being delivered (NMC, 2018).

This chapter will focus on communication with CYP and their families/carers, an essential component for the provision of nursing care to this patient group. The chapter aims to capture this fundamental nursing skill by using authentic clinical scenarios and encouraging you to identify strategies to ensure safe and effective communication. We begin by looking at relevant nursing skills, followed by identifying the possible challenges to effective communication with CYP and their families/carers. The importance of communication within safeguarding issues is also discussed and the chapter ends with focusing on the importance of communication within the muti-disciplinary team who care for sick CYP. It will become clear how having these communication skills ensures that nurses are practising evidence-based care whilst upholding the rights of CYP.

Nursing skills for communicating with CYP and their families

Throughout your nursing training, you will learn about the importance of communication. As well as being a topic taught in your university-based modules, you will also learn from the professionals you work alongside in clinical placement. Showing that you can communicate effectively is also included in your practice assessment documents.

The aims presented within Chapter 1 of this textbook are all relevant to our discussions within this chapter as nursing CYP utilises similar evidence-based practice. This includes the use of generic methods of nursing communication such as completing patient documentation, 'Huddles' and handovers. However, there are additional specific skills needed to communicate with sick CYP and their families/carers, which can differ to caring for other patient groups.

The age of sick CYP ranges from neonates to teenagers, and so nurses need to possess the knowledge and ability to communicate with this entire spectrum of CYP. For each age group, CYP have differing levels of cognitive capability and ability to communicate their thoughts. Therefore, nurses need to be aware of the associated evidence base of communicating with CYP as well as the 'normal' stages of paediatric language development.

Not only do nurses have to be aware of the age and stage of communication of the sick CYP, the family/carers should also be directly involved with any care planning. When caring for sick CYP, the main way to do this is through *family-centred care*. This approach helps acknowledge both CYP and the people who are important to them. Parents of CYP may also need to give permission for medical procedures and so need to have the relevant information to be able to provide informed consent. Nurses must be able to explain treatments, interventions and plans of care to both CYP and their families/carers.

Linda Shields writes regularly about family-centred care and how this can be used in paediatric nursing practice. Shields suggests that *an admitted child can never be treated as a single individual patient, that the family is the unit of care, as the parents and family are central to the child's wellbeing, especially during traumatic experiences* (Shields, 2015, page 139). Effective communication is an essential part of family-centred care to ensure that the views of both the child and those closest to them can be fully acknowledged by nurses (Shields, 2015).

Nurses should especially be mindful of including fathers fully in their communication and care planning. Healthcare teams can often focus most of their communication on mothers, leaving fathers feeling unequal and left out of essential conversations (Cray and Embleton, 2018). This inclusive communication extends to nurses needing to be mindful of non-traditional families/parental teams, for example gay parents and non-maternal parents and carers. By using this open and informative approach involved with family-centred care, trust can be built between nurses and the families/carers of the sick CYP (King, Lacey and Hunt, 2022).

Case study: Luke

Born prematurely this morning, Luke has been admitted to the Special Care Baby Unit (SCBU) for treatment as he is exhibiting signs of respiratory distress. The care plan for Luke will include receiving non-invasive ventilation and being enterally fed via an orogastric tube. Luke's parents, Bob and Marie (who both speak English) are present on the SCBU with Luke and appear very anxious.

Activity 6.1   Decision-making

What actions could the SCBU nurses take to ensure that effective family-centred care is provided for Luke and his parents?

There is an outline answer to this question at the end of the chapter.

Not only do nurses need to explain medical care decisions to maintain family-centred care, these explanations can also assist in *health promotion*. This is another important part of caring for CYP and their families/carers to help prevent CYP becoming unnecessarily unwell. Examples can include community-based activities such as administration of childhood immunisations and thorough discharge planning in the acute setting from hospital to home. Rabbit and Coyne (2012) share the example that nurses have an essential role to play in decreasing the contemporary childhood obesity epidemic in the UK. Nurses need to have the ability to have sensitive discussions with CYP and their families/carers about weight loss and maintaining a healthy diet. Again, nurses need to be informative and to be able to build a relationship with CYP and their families/carers to promote these health promotion discussions.

Scenario: Bradley

You are a first-year student nurse on a two-week placement with the children's community nursing team helping care for 15-year-old Bradley who has had type 1 diabetes for five years. The new care plan is for Bradley to commence using an insulin pump and frequent glucose monitor to help manage his diabetes. The community nursing team are leading on this care, and you observe the team utilising appropriate communication skills to explain the use of these new devices to Bradley and his family. You also observe how the nurses draw upon Bradley's hobby of gaming as a method of encouraging him to convert to using these digital devices.

This scenario complements a section in Chapter 1 within this textbook looking at the use of digital devices in healthcare. When caring for CYP, nurses need to use child friendly communication and ensure that any new medical technology/gadgets are being used safely by the patient and by their families/carers.

Methods of effective nurse communication with CYP and their families/carers

Student nurses will mainly learn how to communicate effectively with sick CYP and their families/carers during their time and experiences in clinical placement. As with all aspects of nursing, there is an evidence base that will underpin your communication practices. For instance, as Dryden and Greenshields (2020) describe, by understanding the stages of CYP cognitive development, nurses can then be informed in their choice of vocabulary and level of detail of any explanations. Lots of useful resources are contained within this textbook that will help build your theoretical understanding of effective communication techniques. Every CYP and their family/carers are unique and will require different approaches to communicating with them. While being a student nurse, it is a good opportunity to develop your methods of individualised communication. You can build your confidence in this nursing skill and ask for feedback on your practice from the registered nurses who you are working alongside. Ask the nurses questions such as, 'did I speak clearly?', 'do you think that the family/carers understood my explanation of their care?'.

Nurses will also care for CYP who require non-verbal or other types of communication techniques. This can include patients with physical disabilities or an impairment with their speaking or hearing. Communication techniques for these patients could include the use of sign language, Makaton or picture cards that the CYP normally use on a daily basis. It is likely that these CYP will be scared when being admitted to hospital and so, by using familiar communication tools, this will help alleviate their concerns while keeping them informed of their care. It is also important for nurses to involve the family/carers where possible in these cases to choose the best communication technique for their child (West et al., 2020). Families/carers will have in-depth knowledge of the CYP's communication preferences, and this involvement will also help nurses maintain a family-centred care approach.

Case study: Abdul

Abdul has severe cerebral palsy and has been admitted to his local general children's ward with pneumonia. Abdul is nine years old and is receiving oxygen therapy and intravenous antibiotics to treat the pneumonia. Abdul does not like having an oxygen mask on his face and has attempted to remove the intravenous cannula in his hand. Abdul's parents have provided the nurses with a picture communication chart to use as Abdul is not able to communicate verbally. Abdul's parents alternate in staying on the ward as they have four other children at home. Both parents speak English.

Activity 6.2   Critical thinking

Describe how the ward nurses could effectively communicate with Abdul and his parents during this admission.

How would the nurses know if these communication strategies had been effective?

There is an outline answer to these questions at the end of the chapter.

Challenges for nurses communicating with CYP and their families

While it is important to communicate with CYP and their families/carers, challenges can occur that can prevent this process from being effective. These potential barriers can occur in all healthcare environments and in the community.

It is useful for nurses to be aware of these challenges so that they can be prepared to attempt to overcome these barriers.

Common barriers to effective communication

Examples of these barriers can include CYP and their families/carers not speaking the same language as the nursing team. Professional interpreters are available and can be used to explain treatment plans to the CYP and their families/carers. Healthcare trusts have access to these interpreters face to face and virtually, for example via telephone or a live online platform.

Nurses should appreciate that not all people communicate in the same way and may not fully understand explanations being given about care planning. Nurses may need to adjust their communication techniques or use of language. This includes using abbreviations such as 'BP' (blood pressure) or 'sats' (oxygen saturation), shortened terms some people may have not heard before and so would not understand what they mean if a nurse were to use them.

Fletcher et al. (2011) share some fundamental verbal and non-verbal communication skills for nurses as described by CYP themselves during their research. Many of these attributes you will already be using in clinical practice but there may be others that you will need to develop during your nurse training. The main recommendations are listed here:

- to smile and be helpful;
- to be friendly, kind and caring;
- to be able to talk and listen;
- to explain what is happening;
- to be an 'expert';
- to be reassuring;
- to be supportive;
- to be approachable;
- to look like a nurse – professional in appearance;
- to communicate age-appropriately;
- to recognise the needs of young people, including 'alone time';
- to promote self-care;
- to be 'cool'.

(Adapted from Fletcher et al., 2011)

As a student nurse, you should also aim to develop your use of child friendly/age-appropriate language to describe specific medical terms to CYP. You may have some experience of this already from working with or having your own children, but you can also observe the healthcare professionals while in clinical placement talking to CYP to understand how this works in nursing practice. You will also see differences in the understanding of CYP and their families/carers of medical terminology depending on whether they have a chronic health disease; acutely unwell CYP and their families/carers may have limited knowledge of medical terms compared to those who access healthcare services regularly.

Case study: Jakub

Five-year-old Jakub is currently an inpatient on a children's ward within a tertiary cardiac hospital. His parents, Zofia and Szymon, are present on the ward, with Jakub being their only child. Jakub has been referred to the hospital after being unwell at home. On investigation at their local general hospital, Jakub has been diagnosed with a heart condition that requires a surgical procedure. The family have recently emigrated to the United Kingdom from Poland and speak limited English.

Activity 6.3   Evidence-based practice and research

- What methods could the nursing team on the ward use to communicate with Jakub and his parents?
- Why is it important that the nurses ensure that these communication methods are effective in this situation?

There is an outline answer to these questions at the end of the chapter.

Dealing with conflict

Unfortunately, sometimes communication between CYP, families/carers and nursing staff can break down due to a conflict situation. Having a sick CYP can be very stressful, which can lead to families/carers becoming angry and upset. When this happens, nurses need to demonstrate empathy and try their best to calm the situation and help the families/carers with any concerns they may have.

This can be challenging, so healthcare trusts offer specific conflict resolution training to all staff, which can be beneficial to your nursing practice. Isangula et al. (2022) agree and suggest that this training for nurses should include practical strategies to help reduce conflict and build therapeutic relationships with parents/carers. Some useful conflict management strategies for nurses are presented below in Table 6.1 which you should aim to use in your everyday care in the clinical environment. As a student nurse, you could also observe nurses or other healthcare professionals dealing with a conflict situation with a CYP and their families/carers. Through this observation, you could learn valuable techniques and phrases that you can then utilise when a similar situation happens again in your future nursing practice.

Table 6.1 Skills for conflict management strategies for nurses (Adapted from Başoğul and Őzgűr, 2016)

Intrapersonal skills	Use empathy and compromise with patients and their families.
Interpersonal skills	Use good interpersonal skills e.g. provide a caring approach, listening to the patient and their families' concerns.
Adaptability	Be adaptable and help provide solutions to conflict rather than being defensive.
Stress management	Keep calm and be aware of your stress levels during conflict situations. If needed, you can ask for help from a colleague.
General mood	Be aware of your general mood during conflict e.g. if you are feeling tired or stressed, acknowledge this as a reason for feeling annoyed about a conflict situation.

Case study: Maria

Ten-month-old Maria became floppy with a high fever today at home and so her parents telephoned 999. An ambulance brought Maria and her parents to their local Accident and Emergency Department where Maria was triaged by a children's nurse immediately on arrival. The medical team decided that Maria should commence a course of intravenous antibiotics and be admitted to the children's ward. It has now been three hours since this decision was made; Maria has had an intravenous cannula inserted but is waiting for a bed to become available on the ward. Maria's parents have now become angry towards their allocated children's nurse, shouting (in English) and demanding to be taken to the ward.

Activity 6.4   Communication

What communication strategies could the children's nurse use for Maria's parents to help diffuse this angry behaviour?

There is an outline answer to this question at the end of the chapter.

The importance of communication in reporting safeguarding cases involving CYP and their families/carers

A significant part of nursing is ensuring that patients are safe from harm and that their voices are heard. Nurses should be advocates, speaking up if they have any queries about care planning decisions or worries about the safety of their patients. When caring for CYP this is applicable to all age ranges and can include raising any suspicions of child abuse. When caring for CYP, safeguarding concerns can also include *child-to-parent abuse,* which can be difficult to recognise but must be reported if suspected by the nursing team.

Sadly, as student nurses, you will come across cases where abuse is suspected, and you need to learn about appropriate communication during safeguarding investigations. This includes practising how to escalate concerns and understanding the importance of documentation in these cases. Writing patient notes is a form of communication and, with safeguarding issues, this documentation must detail exactly what has happened. Nurses need to factually and objectively document their concerns which may include drawings or photographs of any injuries. All conversations with colleagues regarding a safeguarding case also need to be completed including the advice that was given and how this was acted upon by the nurses. It is essential that you become familiar with the communication aspects related to safeguarding concerns during your nurse training, which can be best achieved by working alongside your nurses in clinical practice (Littler, 2019).

Case study: Leiland-James Corkill

In England during May 2022, Laura Castle was jailed for at least 18 years for the murder of one-year-old Leiland-James, who died after suffering catastrophic head injuries. Prosecutors report that Laura, who was in the process of adopting Leiland-James, killed the boy when she lost her temper, suggesting that she smashed the back of his head against a piece of furniture. Upon investigation of the case, it was determined that a lack of information sharing between the agencies involved heavily contributed to the tragic death of Leiland-James. This included the family doctor, Laura's talking therapy practitioners, Laura's gastroenterologist and the associated social workers. Laura had disclosed pertinent information regarding her anger issues and alcoholism to these agencies. However, this critical information was not shared fully and so consequently was not available to Cumbria Council who went on to approve Laura's application for adoption.

Activity 6.5   Leadership and management

If you were caring for a child and were concerned that a parent/carer had potentially dangerous anger issues, how could you effectively communicate these concerns to the nursing team?

There is an outline answer to this question at the end of the chapter.

Unfortunately, safeguarding cases can be a frequent occurrence when nursing CYP and their families/carers and it is essential that nurses can communicate any concerns or associated actions appropriately. As you progress through your nursing career, you will also develop your skills of communicating *with* CYP and their families/carers during safeguarding investigations. You should begin to observe these practices during your time as a student nurse and speak to the registered nurses about the best ways to do this to ensure that your communication remains professional and effective.

Multidisciplinary team working for communicating with CYP and their families

Nurse communication with members of the multidisciplinary team (MDT) is already included within Chapter 5 of this textbook, demonstrating how important this collaborative working approach is to providing effective nursing care. This next section focuses specifically on the perspective of CYP and their families/carers highlighting the specific MDT associated with this patient group. This includes professionals trained to provide specialised paediatric care, who are invaluable colleagues to nurses caring for CYP.

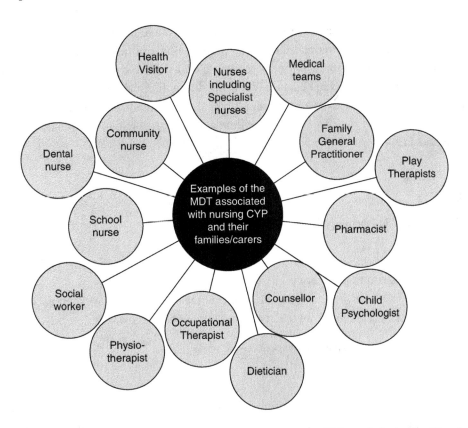

Figure 6.1 Examples of the MDT associated with nursing CYP and their families/carers

As Figure 6.1 suggests, there are many professionals who form the MDT related to caring for CYP and their families/carers. The choice of professional will depend upon the treatment and diagnosis but, ultimately, nursing staff look to involve the expert in their field. This expertise can also extend to involvement with safeguarding investigations whereby the MDT member may have also had concerns, similar to the nursing team, when providing care (Spencer et al., 2019).

MDT working in action for CYP

Nurses may require the help of these specialised professional colleagues when caring for CYP. For example, play therapists are very useful MDT members as they are experts in communicating with CYP of all ages. Play therapists who work within healthcare aim to use play in preparing CYP for procedures and explaining medical conditions (Pérez-Duarte Mendiola, 2022). The nursing team will refer CYP to the play therapist team and should explain why the referral has been made and provide an outline of the health status of the patient.

Case study: Bhabani

The play therapist team in a children's outpatient department are meeting seven-year-old Bhabani today to help overcome her needle phobia. Bhabani has autism and is accompanied by her carer. Bhabani requires regular blood tests due to having a metabolic condition. At present, Bhabani becomes very upset during hospital visits for the blood tests, which results in her carer having to restrain Bhabani during the procedures. It is hoped by the nursing team that the play therapists will be able to assist Bhabani with managing her needle phobia.

Activity 6.6 Team working

- What information should the nurses have given to the play therapists when they referred Bhabani to this service?
- How could the nursing and play therapist teams communicate to keep each other updated about Bhabani's progress regarding her needle phobia?

There is an outline answer to these questions at the end of the chapter.

Nurses should be aware that other members of the MDT may have a slightly different way in communicating patient information; this is a phenomenon that exists in healthcare most likely due to different training and job roles. To overcome this, nurses can use certain tools to streamline their communication with these professionals and use a common vocabulary. A good example of this is the use of the paediatric early warning score (PEWS) systems with medical teams. If the clinical observations of a CYP present outside of the normal expected parameters (lowered heart rate, high breathing rate) then the patient 'triggers' a score of above the normal of zero. You may have used PEWS already in your clinical practice and seen how this shared knowledge of the scoring system can assist the nursing and medical teams in communicating to each other how unwell a CYP has become. When used effectively, PEWS can help the detection and successful reporting of a deteriorating patient thus ensuring appropriate treatment is swiftly administered (Burke, Downey and Almoudaris, 2022).

Another communication tool commonly used in healthcare to aid effective communication between teams, is SBAR. This stands for situation, background, assessment and recommendation. Table 6.2 shows an example of an SBAR communication tool that you can use as a student nurse in clinical practice. Originally founded by the US Navy, this tool has been amended for use in healthcare and advocates the use of a concise method of explaining the status of a patient. SBAR can be used in various patient-related discussions, including

Table 6.2 SBAR communication tool- CYP example for a student nurse (Adapted from NHS England and NHS Improvement, 2021a)

Situation	I am (your name), (X) student nurse on ward (X)
	I am calling about (CYP patient X)
	I am calling because the nurses and I are concerned that... (e.g. BP is low/high, pulse is XX, temperature is XX, PEWS is elevated with a score of XX)
Background	Patient (X) was admitted on (XX date) with... (e.g. febrile convulsion/bronchiolitis)
	They have had (X operation/procedure/investigation)
	Patient (X)'s condition has changed in the last (XX mins) Their last set of observations were (XX)
	Patient (X)'s normal condition is... (e.g. alert/drowsy/confused, pain free)
Assessment	The nurses and I think that the problem is (XXX)
	And my registered nurse and I have... (e.g. given oxygen/analgesia, stopped an intravenous infusion)
	OR
	The nurses and I are not sure what the problem is but patient (X) is deteriorating
	OR
	The nurses and I don't know what's wrong, but we are really worried
Recommendation	The nurses and I need you to...
	Come to see the patient in the next (XX mins)
	AND
	Is there anything the nurses and I need to do in the meantime? (e.g. stop the intravenous fluids/repeat the observations)
	Finally, ask the receiver (the MDT member) to repeat the key information back to you to ensure their understanding of what you have said during your SBAR

MDT meetings, to clarify clinical findings and to make agreed recommendations of care. Evidence suggests that by using the SBAR tool, communication between MDT members can be improved greatly as well as improving the quality of these working relationships (NHS England and NHS Improvement, 2021b).

As a student nurse in an acute clinical placement during your training, you may also be involved with two other specific examples of MDT working and the transition of care to adult services and handover with paediatric clinical retrieval teams. These situations are unique to nursing CYP and their families/carers and so require you to understand the relevant communication involved. This communication includes explaining plans and procedures to the CYP and their families/carers but also professionally conversing with the MDT members involved.

When CYP who have a long-term condition, such as cystic fibrosis or epilepsy, become an adolescent, their care will need to be transferred to the adult healthcare services; this process is called *transition*. Again, nurses will be required to communicate with the CYP and their families/carers as well as the MDT members involved with this transfer of care. Transition should be a positive experience for both CYP and their families/carers as this can be a scary time for them, losing the comfort of knowing the paediatric MDT and clinical environment and having to meet new people in a different clinical area. Nurses and both the MDTs involved need to ensure that at the end of transition, CYP and their families/carers feel fully informed and are able to function in the adult services (Morgan et al., 2022).

Morgan identified some 'Top tips' for MDT communication with young people during transition to adult clinical services. These are:

- Talk to young people in a developmentally appropriate way.
- Use a family-centred care approach.
- Offer peer group support.
- Encourage young people to commence having their clinical appointments without their families/carers present.
- Use motivational interviewing techniques as this is a proven way to talk to young people.
- Always use the young person's name and read their notes before a consultation/ conversation; young people can find being made to repeat their clinical history frustrating.
- Use a readiness tool such as 'ready steady go' (www.readysteadygo.net) as a framework for conversations with young people.

(Adapted from Morgan et al., 2022)

If a CYP admitted to a general ward becomes dangerously unwell, the patient may be collected and transported to a specialist unit in another hospital by the local paediatric clinical retrieval team. This team comprises of highly trained and experienced healthcare professionals including senior nurses, doctors and anaesthetists. As a ward-based student nurse, you will need to learn how to safely hand over to this team ensuring that all relevant information and documentation has been delivered regarding the patient's status and treatment so far. Harte (2022) states that the SBAR tool could be used during this handover from ward nurses to paediatric clinical retrieval teams. Both the ward nurses and the retrieval team must ensure that family-centred care is maintained throughout the retrieval process, before, during and after, in a sensitive but direct manner to reduce the concerns of the CYP and their families/carers (Ford et al., 2018).

Chapter summary

This chapter has demonstrated the importance of communication and also the different aspects of this skill when nursing CYP. The information provided is by no means exhaustive and there is a lot more research and information to read about the topic. The annotated further reading list below, which we hope you will find useful, is a good start to continue your professional development, which we hope you will find useful. Communication is essential in providing safe and effective care and helps ensure a family-centred approach. This way, our unwell CYP and their families/carers can feel valued, listened to and fully involved with clinical decision-making.

Activities: brief outline answers

Activity 6.1   (page 84)

It is important that the SCBU nurses provide family-centred care for Luke, Marie and Bob. Continuous effective communication with Marie and Bob should be maintained to establish a good relationship with the parents and to ensure informed consent for Luke's care. The SCBU nurses should be particularly mindful of the promotion of father involvement as this can be overlooked with the focus usually being on the mother in SCBU.

Activity 6.2   (page 86)

As Abdul is non-verbal, the ward nurses should communicate with him using his picture board. Both parents need to be kept up to date with Abdul's care even if they are not present at the same time on the ward. Therefore, the ward nurses may need to provide a handover to each parent as they visit Abdul. The ward nurses will know if their communication has been effective by Abdul's parents being able to successfully verbalise treatment plans and by expressing satisfaction with Abdul's nursing care.

Activity 6.3   (page 88)

The ward nurses need to enlist the assistance of a verified interpreter to explain the care plan and to answer Zofia, Szymon and Jakub's questions. An interpreter is also essential for obtaining parental consent to the surgical procedure and so that Jakub understands what is going to happen to him during this admission. This is important so that the legally required informed consent can be gained and to maintain a family-centred care approach.

Activity 6.4   (page 89)

Maria's parents are clearly feeling stressed and so are becoming angry towards the staff. The children's nurse allocated to Maria needs to show empathy towards the parents and utilise a compassionate approach in their communication. Talking calmly and listening to the parents will help de-escalate their anger as well as keeping the parents fully informed with regular updates of Maria's care.

Activity 6.5   (page 90)

Safeguarding concerns are never easy to be involved with, but it is essential that nursing staff raise any concerns regarding parental behaviour. In this case, the student nurses may observe a parent or carer shouting or screaming at their child. Any witnessed incidences should be documented and then reported to the nurse in charge and to the safeguarding team within the healthcare organisation.

Activity 6.6   (page 92)

The nurse referral to the play therapists should have been completed as per local policy and have included a clear description of Bhabani's situation, needle phobia and carer involvement. Continuing communication regarding Bhabani's progress with her needle phobia could be maintained via existing MDT meetings and discussions between the nursing team and play therapists. Bhabani's patient notes will also be a useful tool for central documentation of suggested play techniques to be used during her blood tests.

Further reading

Edwards, S and Coyne, I (2019) *A Nurse's Survival Guide to Children's Nursing.* London: Elsevier.

This series of survival guides for nurses are invaluable and this one is specifically for children's nursing. Chapter 5.2 entitled 'Psychosocial Issues' discusses communication with sick CYP and also child protection matters.

Macqueen, S, Bruce, EA, Gibson, F (2012) *The Great Ormond Street Hospital Manual of Children's Nursing Practices.* London: Wiley-Blackwell.

Chapter 7 (child protection) and Chapter 24 (play as a therapeutic tool) are particularly relevant to communication with children, young people and their carers/families in hospital.

Useful websites

helpmegrowmn.org/HMG/DevelopMilestone/CommLangMilestones/index.html

Help Me Grow Minnesota – communication and language milestones. As a student nurse, it is useful for you to understand normal childhood communication stages. This web page lists the expected communication and language milestones.

www.edgehill.ac.uk/departments/academic/health/research/rights-based-standards-for-children-undergoing-clinical-procedures/

Edge Hill University's innovative research on rights-based standards for children undergoing clinical procedures led by support.

www.youtube.com/watch?v=l3CaeyH2GPg

Communicating with children in healthcare | Ausmed Explains...: An informative YouTube video from Ausmed has some top tips on communicating with children, young people and their carers/families in acute care.

www.youtube.com/watch?v=ilZgdu2SbHY

Five effective communications tips for paediatric nurses: YouTube video by The PediNurse useful for student nurses with five top tips for communicating with paediatric patients of all ages in hospital.

www.rcn.org.uk/Professional-Development/publications/safeguarding-children-and-young-people-every-nurses-responsibility-uk-pub-009-507

This document provides practical guidance on the processes for nurses involved with a safeguarding issue concerning a child or young person. It also includes a useful list of resources for further reading around this topic.

Chapter 7   Communication with adults

Naomi Anna Watson

NMC Future Nurse: Standards of Proficiency for Registered Nurses

The following platforms and proficiencies will be covered in this chapter:

Platform 7: Coordinating care

7.5   Understand and recognise the need to respond to the challenges of providing safe, effective and person-centred nursing care for people who have co-morbidities and complex care needs.

7.10 Understand the principles and processes involved in planning and facilitating the safe discharge and transition of people between caseloads, settings and services.

Annexe A: Communication and relationship management skills

2.1   Share information and check understanding about the causes, implications and treatment of a range of common health conditions including anxiety, depression, memory loss, diabetes, dementia, respiratory disease, cardiac disease, neurological disease, cancer, skin problems, immune deficiencies, psychosis, stroke and arthritis.

2.2   Use clear language and appropriate written materials making reasonable adjustments where appropriate in order to optimise people's understanding of what has caused their health condition and the implications of their care and treatment.

2.5   Identify the need for and manage a range of alternative communication techniques.

2.8   Provide information and explanation to people, families and carers and respond to questions about their treatment and care and possible ways of preventing ill health to enhance understanding.

3.2   Motivational interview techniques.

3.4   Talking therapies.

Chapter aims

After reading this chapter, you will be able to:

- define adulthood in the context of human development and models of adult development;
- explain the stages of adult life, events in the lifespan and understand the impact of early adult life events, such as illness, pregnancy, childbirth and parenting;
- explain midlife issues and events (life events) and the Holmes and Rahe 1967 social readjustment scale (Noone, 2017), which rates the stress levels of events such as divorce and other loss;
- outline likely issues that may affect both men and women in terms of overall menopausal impact;
- identify your role as a student nurse and how you may effectively support patients during the various stages of adult life.

Introduction

This chapter will give you the opportunity to consider the stages and experiences of adulthood and the communication skills that are required at each stage. You will explore how specific life events impact on adults at different stages of their lives such as emerging adulthood, adult life and family decisions. You will be asked to consider your role as a nurse of adult patients and how best to apply evidence to your practice.

Adulthood is broadly defined as the period of life where biological, social and psychological changes take place that enable and promote sequenced levels of maturity. This begins at age 18 years and extends through to age 60 years, covering most of active life (Wood et al., 2018). This stage in human development brings with it a definitive process of growth and independence, when an individual becomes responsible for making decisions that will have an effect on the rest of their lives. As a stage in the lifespan, it signals the start of social and physical maturity and intellectual development towards independent thinking.

Being a time of intense developmental activity, it may start with the search for a life occupation or profession and also for a life partner in most cases. Usually, young adults have either made a decision to extend their schooling by going on to university or have gone into the workplace as an apprentice. Others may take time out to travel for adventure before returning to find a partner and settle down. These decisions will all have an impact on how individual lives unfold as they move through young adulthood. Established Adulthood according to other theorists, is the period age 30–45, when major decisions have been made relating to partnering, having children and building family life (Green, 2023).

Models and stages of adult development

Developmental models provide a background to the changes that take place in each individual as they approach adulthood. Brett (2023) identifies Levenson et al.'s classification as a model which has three stages identified as follows:

- Early adulthood: from age 18 to mid-30s. A period that signals emphasis on educational goals.
- Middle stage: From age 35 to age 60: signalling a period when adults look to become married or cohabit, settling down and starting a family/childbearing.
- Late stage from age 60–65 to end of life.

Stage theorists tend to have varied views about how this development occurs and which aspects apply at any particular age in adult life. For example, Kegan (1994) discusses a stage theory model which suggests that adults go through five stages of development that helps individuals to identify the steps required to make decisions about their lives.

These are as follows:

- Stage 1 Early childhood: The impulsive mind; the period which influences how development happens at the next stage, usually from age 5 to 15 years.
- Stage 2 Teen and young adulthood: The imperial mind – expectations of individual needs being met, and rule following is required whether in the home or at school. Keegan suggests that 6 per cent of the adult population could be at this stage, occurring from age 18 to 25 years.
- Stage 3 The socialised mind: 58 per cent of the population.
- Stage 4: Self-authoring mind: 35 per cent of population
- Stage 5: Self-transforming mind: 1 per cent of the population.

Theorists also argue that the stage of development of each individual determines the types of networks that may be necessary in supporting them through important roles such as in education, social and family life and the workplace (Chandler and Kram, 2005). In the context of Erickson's stages of human development, Stage 6 is identified as intimacy versus isolation and include all stages where young adulthood begins at age 18 and lasts until around age 40 years (Dunkel and Harbke, 2017). It is considered to bring with it some measure of conflict and disruption as individuals struggle to shape their futures and establish commitments away from family. Consequently, the success of each individual in this early step of adult independence will depend largely on their earlier childhood experiences and stability or otherwise, of their home life. The task of establishing relationships that are intimate is meant to reduce the feelings of isolation, a not uncommon problem for some young adults (Lim et al., 2019). However, intimacy here does not indicate romance but the urge to form closeness and belonging outside of family context. The scenario below provides an example of a young adult's experience of leaving home and moving to university, while living with asthma as a long-term condition.

Case study: Liang

As a third-year student nurse on a community placement, Melanie's supervisor has invited her into a meeting with Liang, an 18-year-old student whose parents are from Beijing. He is in his first year of studies in electronic engineering at a university. He has lived with asthma as a long-term condition since he was a child. He was referred to the local health centre following discharge from hospital where he had been admitted with an acute asthma attack. He had very recently moved away from his family home to start his university degree. His most recent asthma attack was his third acute hospital admission in less than a month, and his hospital specialist was concerned that he needed support to self-manage his condition more effectively. Liang's GP referred him to the district nurse for a post discharge consultation and the plan is to have a discussion in order to motivate him to take better control of his asthma. At the consultation with the district nurse, Liang says that he keeps forgetting his inhalers in his flat when he goes out to classes and cannot always get back once he has left for the day. He shares a student flat with three other students who are on a different course from him, and he does not get to see them very often as they have different timetables. He also revealed that his flatmates do not include him in their weekend activities and he is feeling isolated, ignored and a little out of place. He had spoken to his parents about his feelings, and they have advised him to move back home. Liang revealed that he does not wish to move back in with his parents but was unsure what to do next.

Activity 7.1   Communication

Thinking about the case study above, and Liang's challenges with his asthma:

1. In what ways could Melanie and her supervisor motivate him to improve his self-management of his asthma?
2. What specific communication skills may be helpful here?
3. Give at least two examples of ways that you, as a student nurse could contribute to the consultation?

There is an outline answer to these questions at the end of the chapter.

Young adults are known to generally want to fit in with their peers. They are usually starting out on many new adventures and tend to be anxious to claim their independence and be accepted. Moving from the parental home to university provides them with what they consider to be a welcoming opportunity to build their own friendships and establish new relationships. Wood et al. (2018) calls this stage emerging adulthood, starting at age 18 years and extending to age 29 years, which can be considered as a critical stage in the development cycle. Individuals are actively pursuing activities to establish themselves, develop a definitive identity and emotional stability in order to move into a settled future. There are many challenges that can affect this stage. Having to live with a long-term condition such as asthma or diabetes, or a critical illness such as cancer, can be quite daunting for everyone, but for young adults, this can be traumatic and debilitating. Mental health challenges are also not uncommon during this stage of life, and it is well known that high rates of suicide of young people is a worrying trend (Arnett et al., 2014). To begin with, some may feel forced to resort back to their parents for support during their illness. Alternatively, they may just simply struggle to accept such a diagnosis and try to manage without any support. This is difficult as it usually means that they have not been able to grasp or recognise the importance of good self-management of their condition. Once they have been identified in the healthcare system following a diagnosis, they will likely need regular and consistent support of nursing staff to encourage and motivate them to follow medical and nursing guidance in order to reduce complications of their illness. Appropriate communication techniques can contribute to the process, including the use of digital apps that young people can access directly from their mobile devices. The use of digital health devices to support patients with long-term health conditions is now encouraged and commonly used. Liang may worry about the stigma of using an inhaler while with his friends. Finding a local or online support network of young persons who live with asthma, or starting one for him, is one way of helping him to cope with his asthma and to live with it without regular disruptions in his university life.

Adult life and events in the lifespan

Case study: Janice and Danny

Janice is 34 years old; she met her partner Danny at university and they got married immediately after completing their degrees. They live with their two children Jamie who is 4 years old, and Sally who is 3 years old. As they were unable to afford a mortgage so soon after university and did not want to wait, they set up home in a flat on the local council estate and both got jobs working locally. Janice worked in the field of cosmetology and Danny got a job with the Charity Commission. When they are at work, both children attend the nursery, and both take it in turns to drop off and collect the children, depending on their shifts. While on a community placement, the student nurse Francis was informed by her supervisor Marion the district nurse, that

(Continued)

(Continued)

a referral had come in from the local Accident and Emergency Department where Jamie, Janice's son, had been treated over the weekend, then sent back home. He had bruises to his face and skin, and a fractured arm. Janice told the doctor that Jamie had fallen down the stairs, broken his arm and bruised his face. Francis attended the visit to Janice's flat with Marion. During the visit, Janice began to cry, saying that she is struggling as her husband has moved out and had asked her for a divorce. The nature of her job involves long hours providing direct care to customers as a beautician. She said she was unable to make ends meet on her salary alone. Her parents live out of town and she has no local support to call on. The nursery won't have Jamie while he is sick, and Janice has to stay home to care for him. Janice confides that she is pregnant with her third child and says she is feeling suicidal and does not know where to turn or what to do. She is thinking of moving closer to her parents; however, she does not know if she will be able to qualify for social housing close enough to them.

Activity 7.2 Team working

1. What are the likely challenges that you and your supervisor could face while visiting Janice?
2. What communication skills will you both need in this situation?
3. Explain the steps you may both be able to take to support Janice as a young single parent.
4. Identify specific members of the interprofessional team who could support Janice through this difficult time.

There is an outline answer to these questions at the end of the chapter.

Life challenges as a young adult can have an enduring impact on patients' lives. Support is a necessary requirement and must be responsive to the needs of the individual. Living with a debilitating illness as a young person can limit them physically, psychologically and socially.

Janice will need extensive support as she attempts to stabilise her life while pregnant and without a partner.

Young adulthood brings expectations of individual needs being met and understanding rule-following behaviour whether at university or in the workplace as a young employee.

Pregnancy, childbirth and parenting: life impact

The Office for National Statistics (ONS, 2021a) state that in the UK, the average age for women to have a child has risen to age 30.5 years. At 34 years old, Janice fits this category having had two children and is expecting a third. Social and family support are vital to ensure emotional health and wellbeing for all parenting families. Some theorists refer to women who leave pregnancy until after age 35 as having a geriatric pregnancy. On the other hand the evidence also asserts that having a baby over the age of 35 has many advantages, such as a higher level of maturity, a more stable career in many instances and a wider social support network. The Health and Retirement Study (Stenholm et al., 2012) which considered maternal age in adult health, noted that effects of likely damage of germ cells in women over the age of 35 years may actually be offset by increased longevity of childbearing women. Additionally, women of this age and above have usually built and settled into a career and may feel much more confident in their parenting ability. Medical and scientific advances also actively reduce the risk of maternal mortality at any age. However, this may not always be the case for women from minority ethnic backgrounds (MBRRACE-UK, 2021). Black women in the UK are five times more likely to die in childbirth than White women, of any age. Possible reasons include inequitable healthcare and access as discussed in Chapter 4 of this book.

Pregnancy and childbirth before 31 years and after 18 years, has always been the recommended timing as the body is considered to be physically at its best for sustaining a pregnancy. However, specific steps are required by women during this time to ensure that the child they are carrying is healthy. For all first-time parents and parents-to-be, the research is now clear that intentional planning to ensure a healthy pregnancy includes being aware of how the use of drugs, alcohol and tobacco, and of environmental factors could negatively affect a pregnancy and its outcome. Communicating with women who are pregnant or planning a pregnancy must include helping them to understand the likely risks and ways to avoid these throughout the pregnancy, especially in the first three months.

Communicating sensitively during pregnancy and childbearing years is an essential aspect of working with adults. It is important to respect individuals' own views about their lives and to provide information that is evidence based and non-judgemental. At some point during your education, you will most likely spend time in a maternity care setting. Working with a patient who is pregnant provides you with an opportunity to influence not just the patient but their wider support network, including their partner, their other children, if they have any, and their extended family members where appropriate. You will need to draw on a range of communication skills with specific emphasis on active listening while respecting individuals as adults and also ensuring that they are provided with clear and accessible information to help them make their own decisions about their health and wellbeing and that of their families. The important requirement is building trust and ensuring confidence in the care being provided.

Janice will need support to set up and attend antenatal sessions so that she can prepare for the arrival of a new baby. However, this can only be initiated after she has had an opportunity to consider what she wishes to do about her pregnancy. As a parent of two other children under five years old, she will need the input of the MDT team to ensure that she gets the required support. Some counselling may be required to help her work through the difficulties that she is facing. Sensitive, responsive and non-judgemental listening skills will be vital, while also ensuring that safeguarding rules and guidelines are followed throughout the process.

Middle age: midlife issues and events

Scenario: Samuel

You are on placement in the GP's surgery with your supervisor, when a patient, 49-year-old Samuel, enters the consulting room and informs his doctor that his 22-year-old son Fred, was tried and found guilty of manslaughter two weeks ago. He was sentenced by the court and will be going to prison for 15 years. He knocked over and killed a child in a road traffic accident and failed to stop. Samuel added that his wife has left him, saying she was unable to cope with the pressures. Samuel said he has been experiencing shortness of breath and palpitations and was worried that he might be having a heart attack. Samuel's father had died of a myocardial infarction (MI) and it was the one year anniversary of his death that day. He was worried that his son's sentence may be triggering his own sickness. An electrocardiogram (ECG) was performed in the surgery and identified Samuel as having irregular readings. Samuel's GP referred him to the local hospital, but he was advised that there was a long waiting list.

Activity 7.3   Critical thinking

- Why is immediate hospital consultation this important?
- Find out about availability of hospital consultations in your area and the length of waiting lists.

There is an outline answer to these questions at the end of the chapter.

During the stage of life referred to as middle age (40 years old extending to 60 years old) most adults who have chosen to do so have raised their families and continue to support children through university and in building their own lives. Life events can have major impact on lifestyles and eventual outcomes. In 1967 psychologists Holmes and Rahe conducted research using the medical records of over 5000 patients (Noone, 2017). The aim was to identify if stressful life events are a direct cause of sickness. They developed a stressful life events tool called the social readjustment rating scale (SRRS) that became a well-known and longstanding tool extensively used to measure the impact of life events on adult development. It is still in use today, supported by further evidence that agrees and supports the theory that life change units (LCUs), as each event was labelled, carried varying weights for stress, and the higher the score, the bigger the weight of the event. These established a link between stressful life events and the risk of becoming ill. The weighting therefore suggests that life transitions have the potential to significantly influence adult life and development.

In the context of impact, Holmes and Rahe rated these events on a scale of 1–100. Where more than one life event is happening at any one time, the suggested rates are added together to identify its true impact.

At the bottom of the scale, they have placed minor violations of the law, such as traffic tickets and major changes in eating habits, at 11, 12 and 15 points, respectively. At the very top of the scale, the death of a spouse has been rated as 100 points. Other major life events listed include divorce at 73 points, spending time in prison at 63 points, major personal injury or illness at 53 points and getting married is listed at 50.

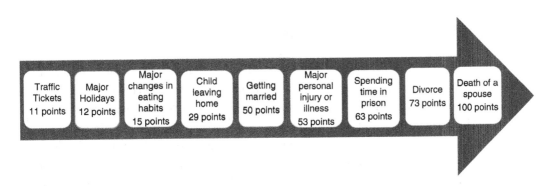

Figure 7.1 Some examples of stressful life events (from Holmes and Rahe, 1967)

A copy of the full inventory is available for individuals to check their own scores on The American Institute of Stress website which has been added to the useful websites section at the end of this chapter. It's important to note, however, that this research was conducted on men only, but it has been widely used for female patients, and is also accepted as having high validity (Noone, 2017). A score of 150 or less, implies a fairly low impact of life events on becoming susceptible to stress, while a score of up to 300 points could indicate a 50 per cent possibility of a major mental health break-down in at least two years' time. Over 300 points signals an 80 per cent possibility, based on the suggested scale.

Menopause as a major life transition

This period of life is a major transition for many women. Historically it is not a stage that has been widely discussed socially. However, this is a common feature of women in midlife and can be very disruptive for many women. The average age for a woman to reach the menopause in the UK is around 51 years.

Menopause, or the time when a woman stops having periods, usually referring to the last menstrual period, is significant not only for women, but also for some transgender men, non-binary people and people with variations in sex characteristics may also experience this. The menopause must be noted as a natural event in the lifespan. Timings and symptoms may vary for individual women. It can also be triggered prematurely by certain illnesses such as cancer treatment or other surgery. In these instances, the onset can be sudden and may be severe.

The changes that take place during this time can have major implications for not only the biological health of women but also their psychological, behavioural and social health. In the UK, more emphasis is now being placed on a better understanding of the effects of the menopause on women, especially in the workplace, in attempts to ensure that there is more support for them during this time.

Case study: Lillian, Tom and the menopause

Lillian is a 55-year-old female who lives with her husband in a small village. Their two children have left home for university and only return at Christmas to visit. Tom, Lilian's husband, works in the city, so is often away for long days. She works full-time in a very demanding job and of late she is feeling unable to cope with it all. She wants to reduce her working week but says she is unable to as she needs the money. At the weekends Tom often goes away with his male friends on his motorbike, leaving Lillian at home alone. Lillian turned up at the GP's office for an appointment with Sally, the district nurse. She complained of feeling depressed and very tired. She had put on a lot of weight and could not seem to shift it, and she just did not feel motivated to try, even though she was feeling ugly and fat. She said she was becoming forgetful as well, sweating profusely and unable to sleep at nights due to the hot flashes, which also affect her in the day. She told the district nurse that she was fed up with her husband, Tom, as he has been leaving her alone at weekends to go off with his friends on long motorbike rides, to which she is not invited. They have not had any intimate sexual relationship for nearly a year, and she thinks that he may be having an affair. He was returning home from his city job very late at night, usually after she had gone to bed. Lillian said she was missing her adult children and feeling overwhelmed by her life. She asked for support to decide about hormone replacement therapy (HRT). She had heard a bit about this on social media and wanted to explore it further.

Activity 7.4   Evidence-based practice and research

What information about midlife transitions for women including the menopause will nursing staff need to be aware of to be able to support Lillian through this stage of her life?

How could you contribute as a student nurse, to shifting the myths about the menopause and attempt to help Lillian deal with her husband's detachment from their relationship?

An outline answer is given at the end of the chapter.

Many companies in the UK are now looking more sensitively at issues of the menopause in the workplace and Lillian may be able to ask for some adjustments in her work pattern.

Specific care pathways that you need to be aware of include those that require a strong level of collaboration with members of the wider MDT as discussed in Chapter 8, and those that provide optimal support in order to maximise adults' opportunities for recovery from illness and major life events, and provide them with the ability to rehabilitate themselves or to adapt as effectively as possible to any ongoing long-term illnesses or disability.

Chapter summary

In this chapter you looked at the way adulthood is defined in the context of human development, models of adult development and an overview of the stages of adult life from varied theoretical perspectives. You also considered the impact of early adult life events, such as illness, pregnancy, childbirth and parenting on the emerging adult stage.

You explored midlife issues and events (life events) and you were introduced to the Holmes and Rahe social readjustment scale and its relationship to stress and related illnesses.

Issues that may affect both men and women in terms of overall menopausal impact were considered, including your role as an adult nurse in the support of patients throughout their lifespan.

You were able to contribute to the clinical outcomes of care for patients throughout the adult development span and apply evidence-based thinking to the concepts covered. You should now be aware that adulthood brings with it a range of development opportunities and is a time of planning and preparing for multiple roles in life including finding one's place in social structures, a job, a partner and settling down to family life with children. This stage can be quite intense for individuals as they progress through the varied stages of roles and

(Continued)

(Continued)

responsibilities, changes and life events even while they are trying to establish their careers and set up homes and raise children. Adults become carers for their children and additionally usually have to also take on caring roles for ageing parents who now need support.

The required skills for you as a student of adult nursing include aspects of not only physical but psychological, social, emotional and spiritual care that you need to be able to use in the support of patients during the varied stages of their adult life. These skills continue to be relevant through the final stage of life, that of old age, which is usually classified as over 65 years old to end of life, covered in Chapter 8. Throughout all the stages of adult life, health education, health support and health interventions as and when required, continue to be important aspects of the care you provide as a registered nurse of adult patients.

Activities: brief outline answers

Activity 7.1   Communication (page 100)

- Your supervisor will need to establish a rapport with him by engaging him in active conversation using open-ended questioning to give him an opportunity to talk about his life and his own feelings about having to live with asthma as a long-term condition. The discussion may well reveal that he had been purposely forgetting his inhaler so as not to feel embarrassed when he is with all his new friends at university.
- You will have done studies on your course about asthma and how it affects young adults. The use of digital technologies to support young adults with athsma is an area you might be informed about. You could contribute by talking to him about his mobile phone use and finding out if there is an appropriate medical app that he could use to support his illness.
- You could encourage him to set up reminders on his phone. You could also suggest that he visits the student union office and asks to be put in touch with groups that support students from minority backgrounds, or with others from his own background since he said that he feels excluded by the students in his flat. He is an electronics engineering student, so he will likely be keen on all things digital. Make sure you are able to discuss this with him. He is also likely to have social media contacts that could serve as support for him at university. You should be able to provide suggestions from your own learning and perhaps experience that can be recommended.

Activity 7.2   Team working (page 102)

1. Janice's children are both under five years old and the visit is intended to not just to check on Jamie's bandage and how he is generally, but to pre-empt the referral to the safeguarding team, as this is potentially a safeguarding issue. You will need to make a careful assessment of Janice's home situation while also assessing her relationship with her children. One major challenge is getting access to the flat to see Janice and the children. Your supervisor had tried to call Janice to prearrange, however, there was no reply. Janice was at home when you both turned up without a prior appointment though. The needs of the children must take priority. A referral will be essential to ensure that due process can be followed.

2. Communication skills required need to not only be sensitive but must use open-ended questions that will help both Janice and the two children to say as much as possible. There may also be a necessity to manage what could be a difficult conversation with Janice while taking steps to ensure that adequate support can be provided for her and the children.

3. Likely support could include further referral to other services such as the heath visitor as both children are under five years old, so that the children can be developmentally assessed and monitored.

4. A social worker can provide long-term support and assist Janice with gaining access to funding and benefits support from the government or from other voluntary organisations. Referral to a safeguarding officer will be required to ensure that the legal duty of responsibilities for the safety and wellbeing of both children are discharged satisfactorily. You have the opportunity to learn from your supervisor and to contribute by sharing information from your studies, for example about local services that may be able to provide support for single parents. Close working here with other members of the multidisciplinary team (MDT) will be necessary to ensure Janice is given all the support she needs.

Activity 7.3   Critical thinking (page 104)

Samuel's GP will need to refer him for specialist care at his local hospital. This is essential to follow up with full investigation so that the problem can be identified and action taken as soon as possible.

Resource allocation continues to be an issue that plagues the NHS. Talk to your supervisor to find out how cardiac care is managed in the NHS trust in which you are a student.

Activity 7.4   Evidence-based practice and research (page 107)

You will need to be able to provide up-to-date information to enable Lillian to make an informed decision about the use of HRT. You could signpost her to online support networks for menopausal women. It may also be helpful to discuss life changes that her husband may be experiencing and how these may be affecting his behaviour. Information on male menopause is now also widely available and may help her to understand some of the problems. You will need active listening skills so she can be reassured that you are hearing and understanding her dilemma. She will need adequate time to explore the issues she is facing.

Further reading

Green, DS, Chuang, SS (2023) Impacts of Religion on Established Adult Women's Lives and Development: Black Jamaican Women's perspectives. *Journal of Adult Development*, 30 (1): 90–105.

Research that explores religion and its impact on established adult women's lives and development from Black Jamaican women's perspectives. This is important culturally specific research with relevance to the UK context.

Springstein, T, Growney, CM, English, T (2022) Supporting Robust Research on Adult Emotional Development by Considering Context. *Psychology and Ageing*, 37 (1): 97–110. doi: /10.1037/pag0000669

Article supporting research methods that encourage an emphasis on context, immediate surroundings, cognitive demands, familiarity, sociocultural and socio-economic influences on adult development to improve research robustness.

Useful websites

www.stress.org/

The American Institute of Stress website.

www.stress.org/holmes-rahe-stress-inventory

Holmes and Rahe stress inventory. Can be used by individuals to measure their own stress responses.

www.nhs.uk/conditions/male-menopause/

Male menopause: NHS England. Provides information about men and the menopause.

www.menopausematters.co.uk/index.php

Menopause support website. A useful source of information on the menopause

www.datadictionary.nhs.uk/nhs_business_definitions/adult_nursing.html?hl=adult%2Cnursing

Gives a brief overview of the role of the adult nurse as described by the NMC and also provides further information of interest in the NHS.

Chapter 8 Communication with older people

Paulette Johnson

(Continued)

Platform 6: Improving safety and quality of care

6.5 Demonstrate the ability to accurately undertake risk assessments in a range of care settings, using a range of contemporary assessment and improvement tools.

6.2 Understand the relationship between safe staffing levels, appropriate skills mix, safety and quality of care, recognising risks to public protection and quality of care, escalating concerns appropriately.

Chapter aims

After reading this chapter, you will be able to:

- understand communication principles as they apply to older people;
- discuss effective communication strategies for engaging with people who live with Alzheimer's and dementia;
- demonstrate sensitivity towards the needs and experiences of older people;
- familiarise yourself with evidence-based and best practice approaches to communicating with older people;
- describe policy perspectives on care delivery, including adult safeguarding.

Introduction

The Centre for Ageing Better produces an annual report entitled The State of Ageing in England; the 2022 report suggests that England is increasingly becoming a challenging country for older people to live in due to rising pensioner poverty and poor health (Centre for Ageing Better, 2022). In 2022 dementia and Alzheimer's was the leading cause of death in England, accounting for 10.8 per cent of all deaths (ONS, 2022a). This fact, along with an increasingly ageing population means it is imperative that health and social care professionals develop the skills necessary to be able to respond to needs related to dementia and Alzheimer's.

In this chapter we discuss dementia (the umbrella term used for a particular set of symptoms). Dementia is not a disease in itself; it is a word used to describe a group of symptoms that occur when an individual's brain cells stop functioning as they usually would. Alzheimer's is the most common form of dementia but there are many other forms of dementia such as vascular dementia, dementia with lewy body symptoms, frontotemporl dementia and posterior cortical atrophy amongst others. An individual living with Alzheimer's disease has a build-up of two proteins called amyloid and tau. Professionals don't yet have a complete understanding of what causes this, but research suggests that the build-up of these proteins causes increasing damage to brain cells over time. This damage affects how the brains work and leads to symptoms of Alzheimer's disease (Alzheimer's Research UK, 2023).

The chapter will provide opportunities to explore how we can effectively communicate with older people, outlining best practice communication strategies for those who live with dementia and Alzheimer's disease. It will also explore the experiences of older people, as well as look at policy perspectives on care delivery and practice at a national and local level. Finally, we will touch on safeguarding policy that provides a framework for improving the quality of care and enabling independence for those who live with dementia and Alzheimer's as well as explore evidence-based practice in working with this group.

Symptoms of dementia and Alzheimer's

The symptoms of dementia include changes in memory, judgement and thinking (impacting cognitive abilities) and also changes in emotions and language (impacting behaviour) (Alzheimer's Research UK, 2022). We'll explore examples of this later in the chapter. It is important to note that an individual can live with more than one type of dementia simultaneously – this is known as a comorbidity, meaning a patient has two or more illnesses present at the same time.

Dementia is a global issue and affects people across the world. The World Health Organization (WHO) reports that worldwide, over 50 million people are diagnosed with dementia, with nearly 10 million new cases reported each year. Age is the highest known risk factor for dementia but it is important to note that dementia does not exclusively affect older people, however, it is one of the main causes of disability amongst older people and places those living with the condition in need of care and support (WHO, 2021a). This data gives as an indication of the prevalence of dementia and the global impact of the condition on healthcare systems, families and individuals. This has led to WHO recognising dementia as a public health priority requiring a global action plan.

So, how do health professionals determine whether someone has dementia? The National Institute for Care Excellence (NICE, 2021) provide professionals with guidance on symptoms which would lead to a diagnosis of dementia: any diagnosis would require impairment in at least two of the following cognitive domains:

- memory – the ability to remember and recall;
- language – the ability to communicate orally;
- behaviour – how a person conducts themselves and behaves towards others;
- visuospatial – visual and spatial perception;
- executive function – skills related to the mental processes that enable us to remember things, focus our attention, multi-task.

As well as this, an assessment should determine whether the individual is experiencing a significant decline in their usual activity or work activity, and the cause of this decline is not attributed to delirium or any other psychiatric disorders. As we are looking at Alzheimer's specifically, we will look at this condition in more detail below. Alzheimer's is a progressive illness so there are early symptoms and symptoms that develop over time as the disease progresses. You will find these listed below:

- Early onset Alzheimer's:
  - memory: forgetting recent events, names and faces;
  - repetition: becoming increasingly repetitive;
  - misplacing things: regularly misplacing things;
  - confusion: not sure of events, times, dates;
  - disorientation: getting lost, particularly in unfamiliar places;
  - language: struggling to find the right words;
  - mood and behaviour: low in mood, anxious or irritable. Loss of self-confidence, showing little interest.
- As Alzheimer's progresses:
  - memory and thinking skills. Impacts on your ability to remember things, making decisions gets worse;
  - communication: speaking and understanding people becomes more difficult;
  - recognition: difficulty recognising household objects or familiar faces;
  - day-to-day tasks: use of basic equipment at home gets harder, i.e. the TV remote control, phone, the kettle;
  - hallucinations and delusions: seeing or hearing things that aren't there, some people may believe things to be true that haven't happened;
  - behaviour: some people become sad, depressed, or frustrated. Anxiety, being fearful and suspicious is also common;
  - physical change: problems walking, becoming unsteady, find swallowing food more difficult, having seizures;
  - care: gradually requiring more help with daily activities like dressing, eating, and using the toilet.

Adapted from Alzheimer's Research UK (2022)

Understanding communication principles as they apply to older people

Effective communication is a key skill required when working to support individuals, particularly when the person receiving help and support is vulnerable and reliant on professional care and support to improve the quality of their life. Dementia and

Alzheimer's can be very debilitating and people living with the condition could be deemed to be vulnerable as a result of the condition and require increasing levels of care and support over time. As a student nurse it is important that you start to develop effective communication skills and understand the range of people you will need to communicate with within your work. This will encompass people of all ages and people with a range of mental, physical, cognitive and behavioural health needs and/or challenges. Communication can take on different forms: this chapter will focus on verbal and non-verbal communication with older people and with professionals.

Activity 8.1   Communication

This activity will help you to think about and develop effective communication skills that you will need to use throughout your work.

Working with one of your peers, allocate five minutes to having a conversation. One of you should take on the role of helper and the other present a topic that they need support with: this can be any kind of help or support. Once you have had the conversation, note what it was that made the conversation effective and make a note of anything that might have limited the effectiveness of the conversation.

Things that you might consider are:

- eye contact;
- body language;
- tone;
- style of questioning;
- did you ask open questions (a question that cannot be responded to with a 'yes' or 'no')?;
- or did you ask closed questions (a question that can be answered with 'yes' or 'no')?

There is an outline answer at the end of the chapter.

The skilled helper model was developed by Gerard Egan (1990) and brings together a range of theories to develop a model that can be used effectively by practitioners from any caring profession. We will go on to look at Egan's work in more detail, but let's start with looking at some of the basic fundamental principles. Egan's model focuses heavily on building relationships with those we are supporting and sets out a very practical framework for *active listening* which uses the acronym SOLER described below. Active listening refers to someone who is actively engaged in a conversation, not only by being present and communicating verbally, but also in their use of body language (Kacperck,1997).

S (Square): Facing the client squarely demonstrates that you are involved in the conversation.

O (Open): Maintaining an open posture is welcoming and engaging. Avoid crossing your arms and legs.

L (Lean): Leaning forward when a person is talking to you shows you are listening to them, you are interested in what they are saying, and that you are involved in the conversation.

E (Eye Contact): Eye contact shows that you are engaged and giving the conversation your full attention.

R (Relax): Staying relaxed for the person you are supporting puts them at ease and demonstrates that you are present in the conversation.

(adapted from Egan (1975))

Activity 8.2   Communication

Using your notes from Activity 8.1, use Egan's framework to make another analysis of your conversation for that activity.

Did you pick up on any of the elements of the model in reflecting on the role of the helper? The SOLER framework is a useful reference for conversations with people you are supporting and for communicating with professionals.

As this activity is based on your own observation, there is no outline answer.

You should now be developing an understanding of what contributes to making communication with others effective. Of course, you will adapt your style of communication depending on who you are communicating with, what the purpose of the conversation is, and what additional needs the person you are communicating with has. Activity 8.1 also demonstrated that communication is not just about your ability to communicate verbally but what is of equal importance is that you reflect on your approach to the conversation and are sensitive to some of the non-verbal cues we exchange during conversations. Jiang (2021) observes that there is increasing evidence that non-verbal cues (those behaviours which are observable but not audible) are particularly important for healthcare professionals working with older adults and can be very relevant for working with people with dementia in terms of predicting behaviour and supporting diagnosis. Below is a list of the types of non-verbal cues that you might have observed during your conversation with your fellow student, although you may well have observed other types of non-verbal cues that are not listed here. It is important to note that non-verbal cues can differ across cultures; what is deemed respectful and socially acceptable can vary across the globe, so considering someone's heritage and asking them what their preferences are is an important part of establishing a positive relationship. Knowing this can also prevent us from making assumptions about an individual based on our experience of their body language and non-verbal cues, or even our own cultural interpretation of what non-verbal cues mean.

Below is a list of non-verbal cues:

- arms crossed on chest;
- hand on cheek;
- head resting in hands;
- rubbing hands;
- tapping or drumming fingers;
- tilting head;
- rubbing eyes;
- rubbing nose;
- tapping feet;
- raising eyebrows;
- shaking head.

Although we should avoid making assumptions about others, some of the above cues can give us an indication of what kind of response we might anticipate in any given situation, or how someone is responding to information or a situation. Where an individual is unable to communicate verbally, non-verbal cues can help to inform their response. Older people may experience changes in communication due to the normal process of ageing, but it also may be the case that communication changes occur because of illnesses that can impede communication. Examples of these are dementia and Alzheimer's and although these conditions are not exclusively associated with older people, they are more common in the ageing population.

This chapter focuses on the older people, but it is important to note that the illness is not exclusive to the older population. There is growing prevalence of young onset dementia (YOD) where an individual experiences the onset of symptoms of dementia before the age of 65, an increasingly common problem due to the increasing population (Draper and Withall, 2016). An individual with YOD might have different care needs to that of an older person and this may require a different approach in how we can best meet their needs. Even if your work in this area is mainly with older people living with dementia, you may well come across individuals with YOD and it is important to understand how the needs for this group might be different in some ways.

Below is a case study that will help you to start thinking about the impact of YOD on the individual and the family.

Case study: Lottie

Lottie is 48 years old and has three children with her partner Sue. They are a same sex couple. Lottie is the main provider in the family and works full-time as a financial analyst. Sue works part-time so she can look after the children and take them to and from school daily. Recently Lottie's manager has raised concerns about Lottie's ability to engage in meetings as she appears to have a significantly shorter attention span. Lottie has worked for the same company for several years and has a track record of being extremely well organised. Recently, it has also become apparent that Lottie is not attending all her scheduled meetings and has not sent advance apologies in many cases. Lottie's colleagues have tried to give her feedback about these changes but when they have tried to do so, Lottie becomes very defensive and has been known to get very frustrated, even quite angry at times. At home Sue has also noticed a difference in Lottie's mood and behaviour. Lottie is becoming very repetitive and struggles to remember significant family events that have happened previously or ones that are approaching. Lottie has visited her GP who referred her to the local memory clinic to access the services of a specialist neurologist. Following a long period of assessment Lottie has received a formal diagnosis of young onset dementia (YOD).

Activity 8.3   Reflection

Read Lottie's case study.

• What issues do you think this family may be facing as a result of Lottie's diagnosis?

As this activity is based on your own observation, there is no outline answer.

Approaches to communication

Communication can be complex and is a skill that we develop over time and with experience. This skill is as important when caring for older people as for any other groups and requires a high level of competence. There is evidence that communication skills can be developed and further enhanced by education and skills training, so it is very important that you understand the fundamental principles of good and effective communication (de Vries, 2013).

We are now going to explore an approach that is considered good practice and where we have some evidence of the effectiveness of the way we approach the task. We referred to Egan's skilled helper model earlier in the book and looked at the practical framework of SOLER, which demonstrates your skills of *active listening*. Egan also developed a structured and solution-focused framework that can be used in different situations to meet individual need for patients with health or social care needs; this model draws on the principles and values of person-centered approaches, in particular those of Carl Rogers (1957).

The skilled helper model works most effectively when the helper (the professional) adopts what is known as Rogerian core conditions of respect, empathy and genuineness (or congruence), using principles of active listening at every stage. Respect involves valuing the patient and having regard for their worth, empathy allows the professional to understand the world and lived experience of the patient and genuineness (or congruence) describes the real and authentic interaction you as a professional should have with the patient. An important part of this approach is *active listening*, which you explored in Activity 8.2. This conveys to the patient that they are important to you and that you are genuinely committed to the working/helping relationship.

Below are the elements of the solution-focused approach:

1. Exploring – what is happening in the patient's life?
2. Identifying aims and goals – what does the patient want or need to change to promote or ensure their wellbeing?
3. Action planning – how could the desired change be achieved?

(Adapted from Egan (1990) skilled helper model)

The approaches and behaviours outlined above are what you could describe as good practice when working with older people. Even the subtleties of the approach will go some way towards ensuring a positive client experience. The next time you meet with your supervisor, you could discuss how Egan's model could be applied in your practice setting.

Diversity and working with older people

Diversity is an important consideration. An individual's identity is multifaceted. It is important to note how an individual identifies can change over time and any one individual has multiple characteristics that make up their identity, which again, are changeable over time. As professionals, it is important that we are respectful towards the people we are supporting and that we avoid making assumptions, ensuring we talk to individuals about their needs and preferences. All public authorities have a duty to think about how their policies and practices affect people, how their decision-making might impact individuals and how we ensure individuals are protected from discrimination. The Equality Act (2010) sets out nine characteristics of an individual's identity protected under the legislation. These are: age, disability, gender reassignment, marriage and civil partnership, pregnancy and maternity, race, religion or belief, sex and sexual orientation. Watson (2019) discusses communication and diversity and recommends the use of person-centred approaches to communicating with older people (an approach that aligns with Egan's model that we discussed earlier); you will have covered person-centred approaches in more detail in Chapter 5. Watson also identifies the things we should be mindful of when working with older people as: not being patronising, maintaining the individual's dignity, having consideration of the diverse needs of individuals, not practising in a way that makes the individual feel fearful or anxious, and embracing diversity.

Health and care professionals have a public sector equality duty not to discriminate against and to provide reasonable adjustments for someone who presents with or discloses that they have a protected characteristic, including a disability. Some older people may present with a disability or comorbidity (dementia plus a physical disability for example). This means that we need to be mindful of our professional obligations and an individual's legal rights. The Equality Act (2010) sets out the requirement of public bodies (including the National Health Service) to provide adaptations that facilitate equitable access to care and treatment. This is an extremely important obligation and not fulfilling this can lead to a breach of the legislation, which in turn has consequences, but most importantly, it can mean that an individual requiring care and support suffers discrimination as a result. To prevent this from happening it is important that an assessment of an individual's needs is thorough and updated as necessary. What should now be apparent is that effective communication skills are crucial in ensuring an individual's needs are met. You will find more information on assessment throughout this book.

As well as our legal obligations, we have a professional and moral obligation to treat others with dignity and respect and not practise in a way that leads to someone being discriminated against. The nursing regulatory body sets out clearly what a nurse's obligation is to maintain professional registration. The Nursing and Midwifery Council (NMC) codes with specific relevance to diversity and respect are:

1.1 Treat people with kindness, respect and compassion.

1.3 Avoid making assumptions and recognise diversity and individual choice.

1.5 Respect and uphold people's human rights.

(Nursing and Midwifery Council, 2018)

Case study: Alphonso

Alphonso is 76 years old and was diagnosed with dementia seven years ago. Alphonso has recently been admitted to hospital and given his circumstances, expects to be in hospital for an extended period. Alphonso identifies as Muslim and while he is in hospital has expressed his commitment to observing his religious practices and, in some instances, will need support with his mobility to do so.

- Alphonso observes regular prayer.
- He has confirmed that he has a halal diet.
- He attends mosque for Friday prayers.

Activity 8.4   Critical thinking

Thinking about Egan's skilled helper model and the NMC codes of practice listed above, describe how you would respond to Alphonso's case.

Think about how you approach your work with Alphonso and what you might need to consider in your approach.

1. How would you address Alphonso?
2. How would you demonstrate respect, empathy and genuineness?
3. What is expected of you from an NMC perspective?

There is an outline answer to these questions at the end of the chapter.

Demonstrate sensitivity towards the experiences of older people

It is important that we are sensitive to the needs of people we are working to support. This sensitivity may relate to social, physical, psychological, or cultural needs of an individual. These may change throughout someone's life cycle so it might be that the person you are caring for is also learning to adjust to a new set of circumstances. We will start by looking at some of the challenges an older person with dementia and Alzheimer's may be experiencing. It's important to note that most disabilities have associated impairments, but each person is an individual and will have their own strengths and weaknesses. It's also true to say that individuals may experience different symptoms at different points throughout living with their condition and this may vary day to day.

At the beginning of the chapter, we looked specifically at symptoms associated with dementia and Alzheimer's. As a professional, you have a legislative obligation to make reasonable adjustments for an individual who has a disability as we have discussed in the section earlier. In relation to communication, this may sometimes be in the form of equipment or aids, so it is important that you are aware of how to use this equipment if you are working with someone who needs this to communicate.

The following activity will help you to think about diversity and accessibility in a clinical setting and how we can respond to the different needs individuals may present with.

> ## Activity 8.5   Reflection
>
> The next time you are in a clinical setting, speak to colleagues to find out what adaptations are in place to facilitate communication between nursing staff and individuals who access the service.
>
> Is there any specific training in place to teach you how to use this equipment should you need to?
>
> If not, speak with your supervisor about how you can get support with learning how to use the equipment available.
>
> *As this activity is based on your own experience, there is no outline answer.*

Making communication accessible

It is important that nursing professionals have an awareness of the range of communication required in the day-to-day role of being a nurse. This will require communication at different levels and potentially to an audience of varied ability. There is a need for nurses to adapt to different circumstances, and there may well be a different type of communication required when liaising with colleagues than you would use to communicate to the people you are supporting. When liaising with colleagues there may be common terminology used that is specific to the setting you are working in, and this may include complex or subject-specific terminology. It is often the case that professionals within a particular setting use acronyms to make communicating more efficient, which might be an appropriate way to communicate if that is the common understanding amongst work colleagues. When you are communicating with the people you are supporting it is important that those individuals understand what you are attempting to communicate to them. It may be that you will need to break down and explain the medical terminology that is used to describe health issues or procedures, or you may need to explain processes within your area of work. Below is good practice guidance from the Nursing and Midwifery Council on how nursing professionals can achieve effective communication:

7.1 Use terms that people in your care, colleagues and the public can understand.

7.2 Take reasonable steps to meet people's language and communication needs, providing, wherever possible, assistance to those who need help to communicate their own or other people's needs.

7.3 Use a range of verbal and non-verbal communication methods, and consider cultural sensitivities, to better understand and respond to people's personal and health needs.

7.4 Check people's understanding from time to time to keep misunderstanding or mistakes to a minimum.

7.5 Be able to communicate clearly and effectively in English.

(NMC, 2018, page 10)

Policy perspectives of care

The National Institute for Care and Excellence (NICE) provides guidance for professionals and the public on good practice, taking account of value for money across the National Health Service and social care. As we've already discussed, people living with dementia will usually need to access both health and social care services as part of a treatment package. You can find more information about how professionals work in multidisciplinary teams in Chapter 5.

Safeguarding vulnerable people is a crucial part of the work we do. When we refer to safeguarding, we are referring to the actions we take to promote the welfare of vulnerable people in order to protect them from harm. An individual's vulnerability may be due to age (in this case older people) mental and/or physical health needs. Across the UK there is different legislation to protect vulnerable groups, but what they all have in common is a framework that exists to protect individuals who are unable to protect themselves.

In England the Care Act (Legislation.gov.uk, 2014a) refers to people with care and support needs. All people who come in to contact with people with care and support needs (who may be vulnerable to abuse and neglect) should understand that safeguarding procedures apply to this group. Under the Care Act (2014a), the level of need is not relevant, and the adult does not have to have eligible needs for care and support from the local authority for safeguarding duties to apply.

In Scotland, a protected adult is defined in Section 94 of the Protection Vulnerable Groups Act (2007 – updated 2016) as an individual aged 16 or over who is provided with/or receives care, support, or a welfare service. 'Protected adult' is a service-based definition that avoids labelling adults on the basis of having a specific condition or disability. There are four categories of services and receipt of any one of these makes an individual a protected adult:

1. registered care services;
2. health services;
3. community care services;
4. welfare services.

(Protection of Vulnerable Groups (Scotland) Act 2007)

In Northern Ireland it is recognised that most adults live independently and free from abuse or harm, however, there are some adults who, because of their situation or circumstances, may be unable to protect themselves from abuse, neglect, or exploitation. The adult safeguarding operational procedures refer to adults at risk of harm and adults in need of protection (RQIA, 2016).

In Wales the Social Services and Well-being (Wales) Act 2014 refers to people with care and support needs who, as a result of these needs, are unable to protect themselves against abuse or neglect or the risk of abuse or neglect (Legislation. gov.uk, 2014b).

Mental capacity also has a legislative framework which is relevant to people living with dementia. As with safeguarding legislation, mental capacity is defined in the context of the devolved nations and has legislation that applies to how this is managed. You will find more detailed discussion about how this legislation is applied in more detail in the chapter on mental health and wellbeing.

Evidence-based and best practice

The NHS provides practical advice on communicating with someone with dementia (NHS, 2023). The advice includes how you as a professional could utilise appropriately any aids that the patient has been provided with, think about the additional time needed for any communication, think about the physical environment the patient is in and whether there are any barriers such as: noise, obstructions, lighting and think about the type of language that is used in communication, which could even involve thinking about using the services of an interpreter.

For each client group that you work with as a nurse there will be good practice guidance available on how you might approach a given situation. This can range from a medical intervention through to how we engage with older people. The Social Care Institute for Excellence (SCIE, 2022b) works to improve the lives of people of all ages, developing good practice guidance/resources and working with organisations to improve and embed working practices. In relation to older people specifically, SCIE acknowledges that social changes have placed health and social care services under extreme pressure, and this has resulted in increasing numbers of patients living with dementia as the population are living longer. They also promote the use of person-centred and asset-based approaches in working with this client group.

Age UK is a charity set up to champion and campaign for the rights of older people in the UK with the aim of supporting the older population to make the most of the later years of their life. Age UK sets out policy positions, undertakes research on a range of matters relating to older people across the UK, and is instrumental in influencing government policy and championing for the rights of the older population, as well as providing crucial advice and guidance on issues such as housing, finance and wellbeing (Age UK, 2019). Given what we know about the predicted increase in the ageing population and the issues of poverty and poor health, the work of Age UK will be crucial in ensuring that the voices of older people are represented. In relation to older people living with dementia specifically, Age UK provides good practical guidance on how we can do this most effectively. In thinking about how we can support any vulnerable individual, a good place to start is to think about the challenges that a patient might be experiencing and then go on to think about how you as a professional can help to mitigate some of those barriers and enable a positive and supportive relationship.

Admiral nurses are specialist dementia nurses who provide care for families affected by all forms of dementia, including Alzheimer's disease. Specially trained as dementia specialists, they manage complex needs, taking account of the situation of the person living with dementia and the people around them. Admiral nurses have specialist training and expertise which allow them to provide advice and guidance to other healthcare professionals and they work across all care settings as well as on the dedicated admiral nurse dementia helpline. This kind of support and advice can help people living with dementia stay independent for longer and support the people caring for them so that they are able to cope with supporting an individual living with dementia. This provides a vital source of support for families living with dementia and is also a useful resource for professionals supporting people living with dementia (Dementia Research UK, 2023).

You now have a broad overview of policy frameworks and the services that are available to support people living with dementia and Alzheimer's. This activity will give you the opportunity to look at these services in your local area.

Scenario: Dementia and Alzheimer's services

You are a student nurse working in your local trust and you have been asked to support the team with onward referral information for people living with dementia and Alzheimer's within the trust and in the community. The department you are working in has asked you to develop a booklet for other students and new members of staff that describes the range of care available to support an individual living with dementia. You have already been introduced to Age UK so you can create a list of services in your own

(Continued)

(Continued)

local area or placement setting, and any national ones, as well as describe what type of services they offer to individuals and families living with dementia. You must also bear in mind that older people may experience difficulties with their health as they get older, but they may also experience wider issues that could have an impact on their health if left unresolved.

At the end of this chapter, you will find ideas about services you might identify.

Chapter summary

This chapter has clarified what constitutes a diagnosis of dementia and Alzheimer's and has given you the opportunity to demonstrate the basic skills of effective communication. Although this chapter relates to older people you will have had the opportunity to learn about YOD and understand some of the issues that apply to an individual and family faced with that kind of situation. The chapter has also covered the legal obligations we hold as professionals and provided guidance on how communicating effectively can prevent discrimination. You should also have a sound understanding of why we have an obligation as professionals to ensure care and support is accessible, and how communication is a key factor in ensuring this. The chapter will have provided you with UK policy frameworks for safeguarding, best practice guidance relating to supporting individuals living with dementia and given you an opportunity to explore services in your local area.

Activities: brief outline answers

Activity 8.1   Communication (page 115)

You will be looking out for the elements of SOLER (as per Egan's model).

You can demonstrate this in several ways including:

- leaning into the conversation and putting yourself at the same level as the patient;
- reacting with positive non-verbal cues such as nodding, smiling and summarising what you can hear;
- reflecting on the patients' feelings;
- clarifying points, asking open-ended questions;
- staying relaxed.

These behaviours all indicate to the patient that you are actively listening.

Activity 8.3   Reflection (page 118)

In a younger family with commitments the impact of YOD may be different including:

- Potential for early retirement based on health status.
- The financial implication of losing Lottie's main income.
- Psychological challenges of coming to grips with cognitive decline.
- Sue and the children may need additional support.
- Sue would potentially become a carer for Lottie depending on how much support is needed.
- Physical consequences of losing independence – not being able to socialise, engage in physical activity.
- Services for dementia might cater more for older people so meeting Lottie's needs might be challenging.

Activity 8.4   Critical thinking (page 121)

1. You would do best to ask Alphonso how he would prefer to be addressed. You might also make a note of this so Alphonso isn't repeatedly asked the same question.

2. Demonstrate respect, empathy and genuineness by:

   - ensuring you are not using patronising terms of endearment;
   - avoiding making assumptions;
   - asking Alphonso how he would like to be addressed; first name, surname, pronouns;
   - ensuring you are taking Alphonso's religious needs into consideration;
   - exploring what it is that Alphonso requires to fulfil his social, religious and care needs;
   - ensuring the environment caters adequately for Alphonso's dietary needs.

3. From an NMC perspective you are expected to

   - 1.1 Treat people with kindness, respect and compassion.
   - 1.3 Avoid making assumptions and recognise diversity and individual choice.
   - 1.5 Respect and uphold people's human rights.

Scenario: Dementia and Alzheimer's services (page 125)

Ideas about services you could identify:

- Do you have a local memory clinic?
- Is there a clinic that has admiral nurses?
- Occupational therapists can advise you on how to maintain skills and live independently for as long as possible.
- Physiotherapists can help with mobility issues.
- Chiropodists can support with foot care.
- Optometrists can support with eyecare and glasses.
- Audiologists can help with hearing and provide support with hearing aids for example.
- Speech and language therapists can support patients with communication.
- Music therapists can provide therapeutic interventions.
- Dentists can help with oral healthcare.

Further reading

Jack, K, Ridley, C and Turner, S (2019) Effective Communication with Older People. *Nursing Older People*, 31 (4): 40–48. Available at: doi.org/10.7748/nop.2019.e1126.

Read more about effective communication with older people.

Pepper, A and Dening, KH (2023) Person-Centred Communication with People with Dementia. *Nursing Older People*, 35 (2): 28–33. Available at: doi.org/10.7748/nop.2023.e1430 (Accessed 15 January 2024).

Read more about person-centered communication with people with dementia.

Useful websites

Learn more about dementia from an international perspective:

www.ageuk.org.uk/information-advice/

Age UK provides services and offers information and advice on age-related issues.

www.nice.org.uk

Guidance from National Institute for Health and Care Excellence (NICE).

www.who.int/news-room/fact-sheets/detail/dementia

World Health Organization dementia fact sheet.

Chapter 9

Mental health, wellbeing and talking therapies: the benefits of effective communication

Naomi Anna Watson

NMC Future Nurse: Standards of Proficiency for Registered Nurses

The following platforms and proficiencies will be covered in this chapter:

Platform 2: Promoting health and preventing ill health

2.7 Understand and explain the contribution of social influences, health literacy, individual circumstances, behavioural lifestyle choices to mental, physical and behavioural health outcomes.

Platform 3: Assessing needs and evaluating care

3.6 Effectively assess a person's capacity to make decisions about their own care and to give or withhold consent.

3.8 Understand and apply the relevant laws about mental capacity for the country in which you are practising when making decisions in relation to people who do not have capacity.

3.9 Recognise and assess people at risk of harm and the situations that may put them at risk, ensuring prompt action is taken to safeguard those who are vulnerable.

3.10 Demonstrate the skills and abilities required to recognise and assess people who show signs of self-harm and/or suicidal ideation.

3.16 Demonstrate knowledge of when and how to refer people safely to other professionals or services for clinical intervention or support.

Platform 4: Providing and evaluating care

4.4 Demonstrate the knowledge and skills required to support people with commonly encountered mental health, behavioural, cognitive and learning challenges, and act as a role model for others in providing high quality nursing interventions to meet people's needs.

(Continued)

(Continued)

4.8   demonstrate the knowledge and skills required to identify and initiate appropriate interventions to support people with commonly encountered symptoms including anxiety, confusion, discomfort and pain.

4.10 Demonstrate the knowledge and ability to respond proactively and promptly to signs of deterioration or distress in mental, physical, cognitive and behavioural health, and use this knowledge to make sound clinical decisions.

Annexe A: Communication and relationship management skills

3   Evidence-based best practice communication skills and approaches for providing therapeutic interventions.

> 3.1   Motivational techniques.
> 3.2   Solution-focused therapy.
> 3.3   Reminiscence therapies.
> 3.4   Talking therapies.
> 3.5   De-escalation strategies and techniques.
> 3.6   Cognitive behaviour therapy techniques.
> 3.8   Distraction and diversion strategies.
> 3.9   Positive behaviour support approaches.

Chapter aims

After reading this chapter, you will be able to:

- define mental health and wellbeing in the context of its likely impact on patients and colleagues;
- explore mental health policy perspectives and how they may be applied to patient experiences;
- understand the benefits of mental health promotion interventions, communication strategies and services that support patients and colleagues;
- examine your personal self-care awareness and your role in ensuring that you are supported and can support others in clinical practice.

Please be aware that the case studies and scenarios detailed in this chapter contain potentially upsetting information for some readers. Please seek support from your university, tutor or supervisor if you are affected by any of the chapter content.

Introduction

Mental health and wellbeing have recently been given a major spotlight specifically following the Covid-19 pandemic and the resultant impact on the lives of individuals and communities globally. In the UK, prominent people such as younger members of the royal family have added their voices in support with the aims of encouraging openness, reducing stigma and increasing public awareness and acceptance of mental health disorders by sharing their own personal experiences. Historically, according to Purtle et al., (2020) the stigma of mental health illness has long been problematic in all social systems globally and is in many ways comparable to the stigma experienced by people who live with a learning disability.

This chapter will provide you with a generic overview where you get an opportunity to consider the benefits of effective communication to the mental health and wellbeing of patients, their carers and families, yourself and your colleagues. It explores ways that you can contribute to this, regardless of the field of nursing that you are pursuing. If your field of nursing is mental health, this chapter provides an introductory approach to your subject that can be further explored and developed as part of your studies.

Defining mental health

The World Health Organization (WHO, 2021b) defines mental health as a state of wellbeing in which an individual not only realises their own abilities but is able to also cope with life's normal stressors and can productively contribute to their community. This is considered to be an important aspect of the rights of every human being; hence it becomes an essential action to not only promote but to also protect and, where possible, to restore everyone's mental wellbeing. The WHO also argues that there is a global requirement that should be addressed by all societies and communities worldwide. Others argue that mental health is not just the absence of mental disorders, as aspects of the WHO definition may imply, since it is integral to everyone's overall health. It is usually also heavily influenced and determined by environmental, biological and socio-economic factors (Misselbrook, 2014). Restoring and promoting mental health where it is possible to do so should be an important aspect of service provision in all social systems. As a student nurse and a qualified practitioner, regardless of your field of practice, it is a requirement that you develop an awareness of your role and responsibilities in supporting patients who may either have a mental disorder or are at risk of developing one (NMC, 2018). A mental disorder, or illness is considered to be a condition that may affect the thoughts, feelings, behaviour or mood of an individual to the extent that it could have a negative impact on their ability to function appropriately and build relationships (Purtle et al., 2020). The case study that follows provides an example of patient impact.

Case study: Jacek

Jacek is 24 years old and lived with his girlfriend Zofia in a flat in a British city. They arrived from Poland together and initially were both happy and contented, having a lot of fun in the city, and saving to get married. They made some friends locally and integrated into their local social scene. Their parents live in Poland, and both planned to visit them as often as they could, with the hope of bringing them over for their wedding, however, things have not worked out. Jacek was only able to find work on an irregular basis since arriving in the UK. Zofia works as a receptionist in a hotel, and initially Jacek worked there too. When Jacek was laid off, however, and had difficulty finding another job, he became anxious, depressed, and began experiencing mood swings. His relationship with Zofia deteriorated as he became more withdrawn, and they started to argue a lot. Soon Zofia asked him to move out of the flat as she was struggling to cope with his mood swings, and this had started to affect her work.

Jacek accused Zofia of having a relationship with someone else and at first refused to move out of the flat that they shared. He began to drink heavily and to occasionally use recreational drugs.

He started complaining to his friend, Yanik, that he was hearing voices telling him that Zofia was seeing someone else although she denied this. He said the voice told him clearly that there was someone else and she wanted her freedom to be with him. Yanik became worried about him and told him to go and see a doctor, but Jacek had not registered with a GP surgery and said that he was fine, he just felt a bit down and would be okay. He eventually moved in with Yanik, but his mood swings became worse.

One night, Jacek woke Yanik up and told him that he had heard the voice again, and that Zofia's new boyfriend was planning to come after him. He asked Yanik to come with him to Zofia's flat to confront her new boyfriend. Yanik refused to go, so Jacek went alone to the flat and began banging on the door and shouting. He shouted to Zofia to come out telling her that he knew she was in there with her new boyfriend. Zofia called the police who arrived, and Jacek was taken to the police station, where he repeated that a voice had told him that Zofia's new boyfriend was out to get him, and he'd had to go to Zofia's flat to confront him. Eventually Jacek was taken by the police first to the station, then to the local psychiatric unit where he was admitted against his wishes, under the Mental Capacity Act (2007) for an assessment.

When he arrived in the unit, he was irritated and upset and smelled strongly of alcohol. He kept saying that his ex-girlfriend and her new boyfriend were out to get him, that a voice had told him and he had to do something about it.

Activity 9.1 Communication

Read Jacek's case study and consider the following questions.

1. Consider Jacek's wellbeing prior to his breakdown. What were the triggers that led to his problems?
2. If you were a student on the psychiatric unit when Jacek was admitted, and your supervisor asked you to come with them to assess him, what would you need to know before his assessment?
3. Outline the likely approach that your supervisor would take with Jacek's assessment.
4. What are the possible communication challenges that you might both encounter and how could these be managed?

There is an outline answer to these questions at the end of the chapter.

Communication with mentally distressed patients can be challenging and unpredictable, especially where a patient's first language is not English or if they have been racialised (Brown, 2003). However, even where patients speak English, the added anxiety created by being unwell may cause behaviour that is not reflective of patients' usual pattern (Carter, 2019). This can vary depending on the type of mental health disorder and how this may have been triggered. Being aware of patients' assessment history and type of disorder provides an initial resource that can form the basis of all intervention. Some common conditions that you may encounter include the following:

*   post traumatic stress disorder (PTSD);
*   generalised anxiety disorder;
*   social anxiety disorder;
*   depression;
*   phobias and obsessive-compulsive disorders (OCD);
*   borderline personality disorder;
*   schizophrenia, which tends to be commonly associated with self-talk and hearing voices;
*   bipolar disorder.

The last three on the above list are considered to be commonly encountered worldwide, however, general anxiety disorder is also widely recognisable in most current social systems.

Do note that self-talk, usually associated with schizophrenia, is generally considered to be healthy normal behaviour that people from all stages of life and positions may at times engage in and may even be encouraged to do in some competitive sports (Galanis et al., 2022). The following scenario will highlight the issues of suicide, self-harm and managing personal wellbeing.

Case study: Phillip

Joe has just started his third-year placement on a psychiatric unit. During the morning handover, his supervisor, Raj, updated him about Phillip, a 20-year-old student who was in his second year at a prestigious nearby university.

Phillip had been on the ward on suicide watch as he was threatening to kill himself and had slashed both his wrists. This was his fourth week on suicide watch. He was observed 24 hours a day and was initially placed in a heavily padded room that was adapted to ensure his safety.

At handover Joe was told that Phillip was taking his prescribed medication under supervision and had responded well to talking therapies and cognitive behaviour therapies (CBT), had slowly begun to open up and was responding to and communicating with staff. Phillip had failed his first-year exams and began suffering with social anxiety disorder and depression and started to self-harm.

As this was approaching the end of his fourth week on suicide watch, the team discussed his progress and decided to gradually reduce his watch from 24 hours to overnight only, 10 p.m.–6 a.m. in his fifth week.

Along with his supervisor, Joe cared for Phillip, engaging him in conversation and in social activities including therapeutic artwork and games. Joe got along well with Phillip and got to know him very quickly. Phillip told Joe that he hated his new environment in the university halls of residence and was not happy there. As Joe was from the same part of the country as Phillip, he was able to relate to him.

In his fifth week, Phillip's suicide watch was partially lifted. He remained chatty and his mood had visibly improved.

One morning, Joe arrived on duty and was told that Phillip had died by suicide the evening before the start of the night watch shift. He was found in one of the toilets, hanged by his neck.

Joe was shocked and very upset and unable to work effectively that day. All staff were distressed and anxious. Joe found it difficult to function that morning, so by 10 a.m. asked his supervisor if he could leave for the day as he felt unwell. Joe returned to work after three days of sickness and requested a session with his supervisor to talk about his care experience with Phillip.

Activity 9.2   Reflection

1. How would Phillip's wellbeing have been assessed while he was an inpatient?
2. What could have been done to support Joe in his care encounter with Phillip? What support should be offered to Joe to help him cope with Phillip's death?
3. Access a wellbeing score chart of your choice online and check your own levels.
4. List some self-care strategies that you could use to support yourself at work in a situation like this.

There is an outline answer to these questions at the end of the chapter.

The increase in suicide and self-harm among young people is now well documented and rising (CYPN, 2022). How individuals are supported throughout adverse life events will play a major role in the way they are able to cope, depending on their life stage, their past experiences and any history of previous mental illness, for example post-traumatic stress disorder. Although measuring wellbeing is subjective, it is one way of assessing how people are impacted by life events as individuals or as a group or cohort (Dolan et al., 2017). The Office for National Statistics (ONS, 2022b) has cited ten domains which measure adult wellbeing. The information is collected across geographical regions in order to assess how individuals and communities are faring across the nations. These include the following:

- personal wellbeing;
- relationships;
- health;
- what we do;
- where we live;
- personal finance;
- economy;
- education and skills;
- governance;
- the environment.

The framework provides a comprehensive overview of adult wellbeing that serves to act as a gauge for likely policy responses within each domain. For example, issues relating to the environment may be influenced by housing and transport concerns. Health-related matters may be impacted by resource restrictions, postcode lotteries or lack of access to healthcare because of large waiting lists. Some of these are major features of post-pandemic pressures and disruptions in health service delivery in the NHS (Hunt, 2022). Applying a national perspective helps to provide a comparison between the UK nations that can assess how different communities are impacted by the above domains. Simons and Baldwin (2021) also add that in an era of post-pandemic chaos and economic fallout, wellbeing emerges as an essential factor when considering impact on the overall mental health of individuals and communities. The ONS has also developed specific domains for UK children and young people (CYP) (Figure 9.1) called 'wellbeing domains' as indicators for the younger population, alongside the adult scale discussed above that can be applied regionally and nationally.

The above scale assesses how children and young people feel about themselves and their lives and is simple to administer. This can be used alongside other assessment tools to enable effective planning of care for admitted patients. It could also be combined with parts of an adult assessment wellbeing scale, which are many and varied. Hospital trusts tend to have their own variations of assessment tools that are used due to the wide variety that is currently available. The Edinburgh wellbeing scale developed by Warwick University in conjunction with Scottish Health Services (Marmara et al., 2022; Blodgett et al., 2022) is widely used across the UK, and is a very popular tool which can be applied to the wellbeing assessment of staff and patients.

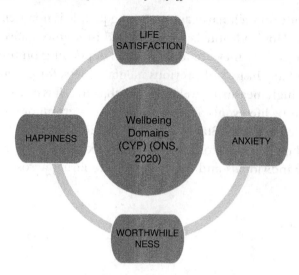

Figure 9.1 Wellbeing domains. Children and young people (CYP)

Although the domains are considered to be subjective, they can be used as a general guide as part of assessment processes and provide practitioners with specific areas of enquiry when caring for patients and their families. This is particularly relevant in an era of post-pandemic recession that impacts all aspects of people's lives and has the potential to erode their state of wellbeing. In turn this can have a negative effect on individuals' overall mental health and that of their families and communities. Talking therapies provide all patients, especially young people, with an opportunity to be heard and listened to. Active compassionate communication skills include motivational approaches, reminiscence therapy and CBT, along with basic skills of non-verbal communication and active listening (Fadipe et al., 2023).

Mental health policy and the impact on patients

Mental health policy in the UK has evolved over time to protect individuals and society, however, many argue that it can also be the cause of some people unfairly losing their liberty without their consent (Blakley et al., 2022, Brown et al., 2023, Brown, 2003). How this is applied will depend on individual experiences, which can vary according to specific incidents in their lives, and in some cases disproportionately so, according to their ethnic background (see Brown, 2003). Jacek was not happy with the decisions that were made, but he was in police custody and they had to act. Note that he was sectioned on arrival on the ward, so he could not discharge himself overnight. In the next case you consider a patient who was compulsorily admitted from the start.

Case study: Sally

Sally is 35 years old and lives with her husband James and their two children, five-year-old Aaron and three-year-old Sheryl in a Welsh village. Sally suffers from schizophrenia and her symptoms have been well controlled with appropriate medication. She worked part-time in a local shop, but she was laid off as a result of the recent pandemic. Sally's husband James became the only working person in the home. This placed a strain on their relationship. Sally began to withdraw, not speaking much and not caring for the home or the children. The school called James to tell him that the children turned up to school one day looking unwashed and had not eaten. The school does not provide breakfast for children. They asked James to make sure the children were dressed properly for school and had something to eat. Sally's most recent psychotic episode was triggered by an argument with her husband who was struggling to provide for the family on one wage. Sally had not bothered to look for another job and had become unmotivated. She spent a lot of time sleeping and took no interest in day-to-day activities. James arrived home from work one evening to find that Sally had not bothered to care for the children that day. He confronted her and demanded that she 'snaps out of it' and start looking after the children. Sally accused James of being evil and of wanting to get rid of her. She told him she had been smelling strange perfume when he comes back from work. She began lashing out at James and shouted at him to get out of the house. She grabbed a knife from the kitchen and used it to chase him out of the house, saying she feels useless and may as well end it for everyone including herself. James ran out of the house and immediately called the emergency services telling them that his wife was in a mental health crisis and the family were being threatened. The police and ambulance services arrived at the house. They were able to calm Sally down enough to take her to the A&E Department where she was sectioned and eventually transferred to the psychiatric unit. It transpired that Sally had not been taking her prescribed medications. She told the team that she keeps forgetting to take them.

Activity 9.3   Team working

1. The A&E Department received a call from the police and ambulance services to say that Sally, who is a patient known to them, was in a crisis and needed to be admitted and sectioned. The case was allocated to Malik, the mental health nurse who was supervising student nurse Belinda on his shift that day. Imagine that you are Belinda: what will be the immediate priorities for both of you when meeting Sally when she arrives?
2. How will your communication skills assist you when talking to Sally?
3. How does the Mental Health Act (1983/2005/2007) apply in this situation? Is this applicable in Wales?
4. What other support will be required by Sally and family?

There is an outline answer to these questions at the end of the chapter.

The purpose of mental health legislation is to ensure that patients with a mental health disorder are appropriately assessed, treated and their rights upheld at all times. In order of timeline the relevant ones are shown in Figure 9.2.

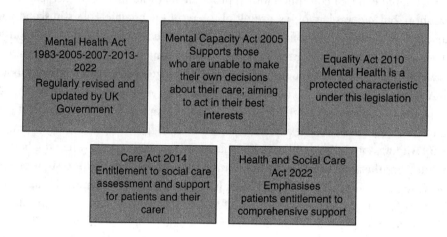

Figure 9.2   Mental health legislation

Mental health promotion

Promoting the mental health of individuals and communities is an essential requirement to enhance wellbeing for everyone. There are a variety of approaches that can directly improve the quality of life for all individuals and communities. Wilkinson and Maurimootoo (2001) identified some of the strategies as follows:

- Ensuring that the capacity of individuals can be strengthened to improve their self-esteem, deal with emotional challenges, improve and enhance their life skills and develop coping mechanisms.
- Work with communities to enable and develop strategies that will assist the wellbeing of the community in the areas, for example, of influencing policy development and of ensuring the availability of skills and training to enable access to work and to self-improvement.
- Removal of barriers and promotion of inclusive practices across social structures such as service access that encourages and acknowledges capacity and rights of individuals and groups.
- Providing interventions that ensure that physical illnesses do not cause a deterioration of patients', carers' and families' mental health.

In the next scenario you explore how this may be approached to support you and your peers.

Scenario: Lillian

You are on a large medical unit, in the final year of your course and in your third week of placement. Lillian is a first-year student nurse on the first day of her second placement. Her first was on a small day care unit. John, your supervisor, asked you to look after her and ensure that she settled into the ward routine. Lillian confided in you that she was scared and worried about this placement as it was such a large ward, and she felt out of her depth. As you were showing her around, a patient whom you had previously cared for collapsed and John shouted to you for help. You left Lillian while you hurried to help resuscitate the patient. Lillian retreated to the nurses' station as she didn't know what to do. Unfortunately, the patient did not recover from the cardiac arrest despite attempted defibrillation by the medical team. You were very upset as you knew the patient well, so asked to be sent home.

The next day when you returned to duty, you were told that Lillian also went home but had not returned to duty.

Activity 9.4   Leadership and management

1. In what ways could you have supported Lillian more effectively?
2. What specific skills would have helped in this scenario?
3. What steps will you be able to take to further support Lillian going forward?
4. Thinking about your own wellbeing, what can you do to strengthen your own mental health in difficult circumstances?

There is an outline answer to these questions at the end of the chapter.

As a final year student nurse, it is assumed that you have experience of ward environments and clinical practice to be able to support a more junior member of staff. Your code of practice expects you to be able to do this (NMC, 2018). It is understandable that in stressful events on the ward, individuals may not always act in the most effective way. Going forward, an action plan may be helpful to prepare you for adverse ward situations.

Chapter summary

In this chapter you looked at the benefits of effective communication as it applies to supporting the mental health and wellbeing of patients, staff, colleagues and yourself. You discussed the use and application of talking therapies and ways that these may be used to enable and improve mental health and wellbeing. You explored opportunities to examine your personal self-care strategies, wellbeing and resilience. Mental health and wellbeing form the cornerstone of effective participation and contribution in all societies. It is important that as a student nurse and qualified practitioner, you develop the required skills and knowledge to support yourself and your colleagues, as well as your patients, carers and families in the workplace.

Activities: brief outline answers

Activity 9.1   Communication (page 133)

- Jacek was a happy and contented young man, doing things all young people do, making friends, and committing to a steady relationship with his girlfriend. In terms of wellbeing, he could be described as having a measure of life satisfaction, commensurate with his lifespan, presenting as a well-adjusted person engaging in normal daily activities. Initially his anxiety levels were normal, his happiness levels high, his life satisfaction and worthwhileness contributing to his adjustment to daily living (ONS, 2021b, page 1). Jacek's problems obviously started when he lost his job at the hotel and began struggling to find work. With only Zofia's salary contributing to the upkeep of the flat in which they lived, and in providing food for both of them, their wedding plans would have had to be placed on hold. These issues provided major triggers that increased his anxiety levels. These are caused by social and environmental stressors that are exaggerated by individual responses such as the use of alcohol and drugs for coping, making the problems more complex (Affengruber et al., 2023, Purtle et al., 2020).
- You would have had an opportunity to listen to the handover report on this patient, which is an important first step in learning about his problems. You can follow this up by asking your supervisor permission to have a look at any records.
- As someone who is most likely trained in the care of patients with mental health disorders, John will be working with specific assessment tools to facilitate this process. These could vary with each NHS trust and across regions and nations. For example, some trusts may have an in-house general health questionnaire (GHQ), a patient health questionnaire for depression (PHQ), a depression, anxiety and stress scale (DASS-21), an insomnia severity index (ISI). The type of mental disorder will determine the assessment process, and you will need to become familiar with the ones in your trust.
- Communication challenges that you and your supervisor may face will be driven by the patient and the circumstances surrounding his admission. Jacek is Polish so it will be important to determine his level of understanding of English. Some patients who are mentally distressed may revert to their first language even if they speak English to a good standard. Applying the techniques and skills covered in this book will help you to become more confident.

Activity 9.2   Reflection (page 134)

1. Wellbeing assessment may vary depending on the NHS trust that you work in. Ask your supervisor about the tools that would be used.

2. In a situation like Joe's, you should explore your feelings with your supervisor. This will help you as you shape your future practice by considering how you may support the students

you will be asked to supervise in the future. Discuss with your supervisor and your peers, using a reflection model such as Gibbs (2013).

3. You have a choice of several wellbeing scales that can be applied to assess your own wellbeing. Most are free if they are being used individually, choose one that works best for you.

4. There are many self-care strategies that can support you in the workplace. For example, learning how to say no, knowing how to effectively challenge others, learning how to have difficult conversations, recognising your own vulnerability (Sellman, 2011) and building your confidence to speak up when required.

Activity 9.3 Team working (page 137)

Immediate priorities are to:

- Access Sally's records, with permission, to update yourself on her history.
- Talk to John quickly if possible about schizophrenia and detention under the Mental Health Act (2007) and Mental Capacity Act (2005).
- Listen carefully to John and draw on your experiences of therapeutic communication.
- Sectioning under the Mental Health Act (2007) involves being admitted for assessment and possible treatment whether or not the patient agrees with the decision. The decision must be made by two doctors, one of whom must be a specialist for the purpose of the legal status. The length of time that patient can be detained will vary depending on the assessment and treatment requirements. Section 2 of the Act allows detention for up to 28 days without renewal. During this time, patients can be fully assessed. This Act applies in Wales and England. Note there are variations for Scotland and Northern Ireland.
- Section 3 of the Act allows detention for a period of up to six months during which time a patient can be assessed, and treatment started if required (Blakley et al., 2023, Brown, 2003).
- Sally has two children, and her husband works as the only income provider in the family. Interagency support will be vital to ensure that the family receives help where required. The multidisciplinary team (MDT see Chapter 5), can provide essential support for this family. Sally may already have a key worker and a social worker. She may also have a psychotherapist/psychologist who has worked with her previously. At some point the team will need to call an MDT case meeting to discuss Sally's situation and make recommendations about her care going forward.

Activity 9.4 Leadership and management (page 139)

- Talk to Lillian after the incident and find out how she felt at the time. Sensitive, reassuring communication will recognise that she is a new student to the environment.
- Arrange a session to debrief her and go over the events of the day and ways to move forward.
- Speak to your supervisor and share your feelings about the events. Recognise your own strengths and limitations and how you may better develop leadership skills for emergency ward situations in future.

Further reading

Barnett, P, et al (2019) Ethnic Variations in Compulsory Detention under the Mental Health Act: A Systematic Review and Meta-Analysis of International Data. *The Lancet Psychiatry*, 6 (4): 305–317.

Reviews and analyses the literature relating to ethnicity and compulsory detention under the Mental Health Act, emphasising evidence-based perspectives.

Jones, K (2023) *A History of the Mental Health Services*. Abingdon: Taylor & Francis.

Provides an historical overview of mental health services.

Zigmond, T and Brindle, N (2022) *A Clinician's Brief Guide to the Mental Health Act.* Cambridge: Cambridge University Press.

A quick access guide to the Mental Health Act for practitioners.

Useful websites

https://www.gov.wales/mental-health-strategy

The Mental Health Act (1983) is the main piece of legislation that covers the assessment, treatment and rights of people with a mental health disorder in Wales and England.

westerntrust.hscni.net/about-the-trust/mental-capacity-act/

The Mental Capacity Act (Northern Ireland) 2016 provides a statutory framework for people who lack capacity to make a decision for themselves and for those who now have capacity but wish to make preparations for a time in the future when they lack capacity.

www.mwcscot.org.uk/law-and-rights/mental-health-act

Covers the care of Scottish people with a mental disorder, defined under the Act to include any mental illness, personality disorder or learning disability.

www.nhs.uk/mental-health/social-care-and-your-rights/mental-health-and-the-law/ mental-health-act/

The Mental Health Act (1983) regulates compulsory detention and treatment of people with a mental disorder in England and Wales. Updated by The UK Parliament on 11 May 2023.

www.mentalhealth.org.uk/

A UK charity with a mission to help people understand, protect and sustain their mental health.

www.mind.org.uk/

One of the oldest mental health charities in the UK, MIND provides advice and support in order to empower and enable those who experience mental health problems.

warwick.ac.uk/fac/sci/med/research/platform/wemwbs/

The Warwick-Edinburgh mental wellbeing scale (WEMWBS) is a scale of 14 positively worded items for assessing a population's mental wellbeing.

Chapter 10   Communication with people who live with learning disabilities

Naomi Anna Watson

NMC Future Nurse: Standards of Proficiency for Registered Nurses

The following platforms and proficiencies will be covered in this chapter:

Platform 1: Being an accountable professional

1.7   Demonstrate understanding of research methods, ethics and governance in order to critically analyse, safely use, share and apply research findings to promote and inform best nursing practice.

Platform 2: Promoting health and preventing ill health

2.3   Understand the factors that could lead to inequalities in health outcomes.

2.9   Use appropriate communication skills and strengths-based approaches to support and enable people to make informed choices about their care to manage health challenges in order to have satisfying and fulfilling lives within the limitations caused by reduced capability, ill health and disability.

Annexe A: Communication and relationship management skills

4.2.3 A calm presence when dealing with conflict.

4.24 Appropriate and effective confrontation strategies.

4.2.5 De-escalation strategies and techniques when dealing with conflict.

Chapter aims

After reading this chapter, you will be able to:

- define disability, in the context of its individual impact and social implications;
- explain the historical context of disability generally and learning disability specifically, from UK perspectives and how this was eventually influenced by legislation and policy;

(Continued)

(Continued)

- discuss a range of models of disability and their application to people's lives;
- understand challenging behaviours of those who live with learning disability and consider how a strengths-based approach may support them to live independently.

Introduction

In this chapter you explore issues relating to disability generally and learning disability specifically, the historical perceptions, types of disability and the ways in which the lives of individuals have been impacted through living with a disability, whether physical, learning, or both. You also consider legal and policy perspectives, lived experiences, models of disability and communication strategies that could support your practice as a student nurse. The chapter provides an overview for nurses preparing for the adult field. If your field of nursing is learning disability, it will give you a general introduction to your subject that must be further explored and developed in depth as part of your studies.

Definitions

The Equality Act (2010) defines disability as a physical or mental impairment that causes substantial long-term effects on an individual's activities of daily living. Additionally, MENCAP, an organisation that supports people who live with a learning disability (LD), defines the condition as 'reduced intellectual ability and difficulty with everyday activities, such as household tasks, socialising or managing money, which affects their whole lives. It often at times may mean that they also take a bit longer to learn and could need extra support to develop new skills, and understand complicated information, learn new things, and interact with people' (MENCAP, n.d).

Causes

Although the cause is not known for many who live with LD (Gottlieb, 2012) some possibilities include the following:

- Hereditary and genetic factors, for example, Down's syndrome.
- Brain injury or damage caused at birth, from traumatic delivery or oxygen deficiency in the womb, likely to lead to mild moderate or even severe LD.
- Brain damage before birth caused by, for example infections such as rubella, or drug and alcohol use and abuse.

The following scenario outlines an example from the experience of someone who lives with complex needs.

Scenario: Carmen

Carmen is 24 years old and lives with Down's syndrome (trisomy 21), a genetic condition, which causes mild to moderate intellectual disability. She has a congenital heart defect and has type 1 diabetes for which she has insulin injections. She also has a hearing impairment and wears a hearing aid. Carmen lives at home with her parents Milly and Frank, and is supported by a key worker Jonathan, who visits her regularly. She works part-time in the local newsagent shop. Carmen was admitted to your ward (a medical diabetic unit) to stabilise her diabetes and has been on sliding scale insulin since her arrival. Her boyfriend Simon, who also lives with Down's syndrome, tried to visit her alone while she was in hospital. On his first visit, however, he was not allowed in, because the staff said he needed permission from her parents. However, neither Carmen nor her key worker Jonathan were consulted. Following the handover session on your first placement, your supervisor asked you to talk to Carmen to find out if she wishes to see Simon and whether her parents are aware of their relationship. Carmen was upset and angry, saying that she does not need her parent's permission to see her boyfriend and she doesn't know why they are refusing to let him in to visit her. You report back to your supervisor who says that it's best to wait until her parents arrive to find out if they are aware of her relationship with Simon. You return to tell Carmen who started crying. She then told you that she wishes to discharge herself from the hospital as she is not happy on your ward.

Activity 10.1 Critical thinking

Read Carmen's scenario above and consider the following questions:

1. Outline an alternative approach that could be taken by hospital staff in this case.
2. What communication skills will you need to be able to support Carmen?
3. Find out what services are provided on a medical ward to support patients who live with a learning disability when they are admitted and throughout their stay.

There is an outline answer to these questions at the end of the chapter.

Those who live with two or more disabilities may experience more life challenges, making it difficult to not only live independently, but to communicate. They will need higher levels of support and multiple interventions, however, this will always vary depending on the type and the complexity of problems. Despite many likely issues, people who live with Down's syndrome can live independently with appropriate support. Carmen lives with complex disabilities so her needs must be carefully assessed to ensure that she receives the right amount of support to enable her to function independently (Brady et al., 2023). It is important that she is treated with respect and recognition of her strengths (Baum et al., 2023). Finding out about individual variations of this condition through an individual assessment process should help to ensure that the right support can be provided.

Contextual and historical approaches

Representation of disability in general and of learning disability specifically has a long history of negativity both in the UK and globally. This has had a major impact on the way that people who lived with any disability were perceived and treated. Going back to the eighteenth century, having a disability carried with it a number of negative connotations based on religious beliefs and superstitious myths. These blamed mothers for acts of sin as a causative factor along with viewing a disabled person or other 'strange images' during early pregnancy, which would allegedly cause the foetus to also be disabled. Additionally, there existed a belief that having to accept a disability involved bearing one's lot in life with humility, not complaining and accepting things as they were (Hughes et al., 2017). These widely held social beliefs led to disabled people being housed away from mainstream communities in large institutions which separated them from the rest of society, essentially hiding them away in large asylums. However, those who lived with dwarfism were used as circus clowns or sometimes hired out to entertainers, simply to be made fun of in society.

Shifting perceptions

These enduring attitudes persisted well into the twenty-first century, until an overall shift was triggered by policy and disability legislation, discussed later. The Thalidomide scandal that took place in the 1960s, also contributed as a factor, prompting a major discourse and national debate and bringing the disability issue under the public spotlight (*The Guardian*, 2012). It resulted not only in the eventual withdrawal of the Thalidomide drug for the treatment of morning sickness but in wider discussions about the care of disabled people in society. The Thalidomide drug is still used to treat some conditions but is strictly monitored whenever it is recommended in treatment of any patients, especially women of childbearing age. Consider below the case of Jimmy, who lives with dwarfism.

Case study: Jimmy

Jimmy is 50 years old. He lives alone quite near to his parents. Jimmy's mother was given the Thalidomide drug during early pregnancy, and she also caught rubella infection during the early months of her pregnancy, resulting in him also becoming infected with the rubella virus. This left him living with a mild learning disability alongside his dwarfism, making him physically and learning disabled. Although Jimmy takes time to learn and grasp concepts, he is able to make himself understood.

Jimmy could get around without much difficulty, except initially where access was difficult due to his short stature. His parents and his key worker Daniel supported him to get his flat adapted so he could use facilities such as the bath, kitchen and cupboards.

Jimmy was admitted to the unit for a surgical operation to remove his gall bladder. He would need support to be able to use regular hospital facilities as he is only three feet tall with very short arms and legs. His parents, who live near his flat, came with him to the hospital. Jimmy was placed in a side room that had a high bed that he could not get into without help. The sink was also too high in the room, so he had to stretch to access the tap. Jimmy was shown the toilet and again, access was not possible. His parents asked for a meeting with Sheila, the ward manager, to complain on Jimmy's behalf that the space that Jimmy had to use while he was on the ward had not been appropriately prepared or adapted for his use, and he would struggle as an inpatient. The hospital was aware of his planned admission prior to him arriving and his parents were upset that no one seemed to have done anything to get the space ready for his arrival. They wanted to know how he was going to be supported before and after his operation.

Activity 10.2   Decision-making

1. Find out about facilities and resources that are available on a surgical ward to support patients with a physical or learning disability, or both.
2. Is required support in a surgical ward environment a realistic expectation for patients who live with a physical or learning disability or both? Look this up on the trust's intranet pages.
3. What communication skills would you find useful in this instance, to work with Jimmy and his family?
4. What is the relevance of legislative policy in these instances, and can they be applied here?

There is an outline answer to these questions at the end of the chapter.

Policy and legislation have one primary purpose, which is to enable people who live with LD to be supported to live their best life, free from discrimination. The main statutory frameworks for you to explore further include the following:

- the Disability Discrimination Act (DDA) 2005 (Legislation.gov.uk, 2005a), which updated the 1995 legislation;
- the Mental Capacity Act (MCA) 2005 (Legislation.gov.uk, 2005b), which also applies to those who live with a mental disorder and aims to protect those who are vulnerable and unable to make their own decisions;

- the Equality Act (2010), which replaced the DDA (Legislation.gov.uk, 2010) as an overarching policy with nine protected characteristics, including disability;
- the Health and Social Care Act (Legislation.gov.uk, 2022) is an act that aims to tackle health inequalities in the NHS and ensure improved health and social care outcomes for everyone, including those who are vulnerable.

People who live with a learning disability require skilled communication techniques to support them in their daily lives and their attempts to access services. Lewis et al. (2017) noted that nurses in some clinical environments feel unprepared to care for LD patients. An understanding of the varied support networks that they may need to call on at some point is one way of overcoming this issue. Communication aids include, for example, the Makaton system, the sign-along system and the British sign language (BSL) system. Jimmy's admission into an ordinary ward for a routine operation will present a number of challenges that can be addressed, even before he arrives on the ward. The Equality Act (2010) makes this a requirement.

Models of disability and their application

Models of LD are widely used to provide a framework to understanding the continuous shift in social attitudes. Goldiner (2022) identifies, analyses and compares six models. However, here we focus on the four main ones that have shaped the discourse and trajectories of the lives of those who live with LD, relevant to this book. They are the:

- medical model;
- social model;
- resistance model;
- affirmation model.

Medical model

Historically, society initially treated all forms of disability, including learning disability, from a medical perspective only, which sits within a paradigm of biological construct. Medical models of health tend to be fixated on identifying the causal factors of disease process and application of treatment in an attempt to cure the problem, so 'cure' rather than 'care' was always given the emphasis. In the context of disability, the medical model therefore works from the assumption that individuals are disabled because of a causal factor or an impairment, hence the issue is personal to them (Brisenden, 1986, Bunbury, 2019).

Social model

The social model of disability, however, begins from the assumption that it is social barriers and structures, created in our environment that impede the lives of disabled people. If these barriers are removed, it is possible for all disabled people to live like 'normal' people in society (Lawson and Beckett, 2021; Giri et al., 2022). The model was created by disabled people as a way of challenging the status quo and removing the burden of guilt and responsibility from them. For example, a building without ramps is a structural barrier to people who use a wheelchair. UK law now dictates that all public buildings should provide wheelchair access and must use a loop system for people who use a hearing aid. For those who support this model, disability is exaggerated by these structural barriers that disadvantage disabled people. An impairment is the actual experience of a functional problem such as hearing loss, which requires sound to be louder so people can hear.

Resistance model

The resistance model of disability builds on the concepts of the social model and works to encourage and enable disabled people to take personal action to resist the oppressive structural and attitudinal processes that limit their life experience (Beresford, 2020). This could be by refusing to be labelled by the social terms that are used to define them. For example, the term 'enabled' is considered a term that disabled people prefer to use to define themselves, rather than the term 'disabled', which is commonly engrained in our social systems (Brady and Franklin, 2023).

Affirmation model

The affirmation model supports the social and resistance models, and places specific emphasis on outcomes that are positive, rather than on negative problems. The assumption is always that everyone with an LD can lead an improved life with the right attitudinal, physical and social support. Emphasis is on living their lives to the fullest, by taking back control, rather than on the actual disability. Individuals are enabled towards self-empowerment, positive identity and improved self-esteem (Flynn, 2022, Chordiya et al., 2023).

The case study that follows gives you an opportunity to explore their application in people's lived experience.

Case study: Toby and Mandy

Toby is 20 years old and lives with his parents, Mark and Debbie, and his younger sister Jane. His mother Debbie had an instrumental delivery during his birth, when forceps were used to rotate his head due to its posterior position in the birth canal.

Toby's development was slow as a child, and he was not able to reach all of his developmental milestones. His speech is slurred, and his physical movements are exaggerated. He was eventually diagnosed as learning disabled. Toby's parents have been his main carers for all his life, and

(Continued)

(Continued)

they are very protective of him. They decided not to send him into residential care or to a school for special educational needs. Instead, they tried to keep him in their local mainstream school. However, this was a challenge for the school and for the family, especially Jane, Toby's younger sister, who is 15 years old. Jane is embarrassed by Toby and upset that he gets so much attention at home and at school, while her needs are often ignored. She is struggling with her GCSEs and her grades have been dropping. As Toby moves into adulthood, his behaviours have become more challenging, and he is questioning his parents more about the decisions they have been making for him each day. The family are having difficulties managing his care. They went to their GP to ask for support, but made it clear they did not wish to send him away.

The family was offered day services and Toby was sent to a local activity centre where he was able to socialise and learn with peers.

At the centre Toby met Mandy, who is 19 years old. She is on her GP's LD register and has been going to the centre for some time. Mandy and Toby became great friends and started spending a lot of time in each other's company.

Toby's parents were relieved that he had settled so well in the new day centre and was enjoying his time there but were anxious about his developing relationship with Mandy and spoke to the centre manager about putting them in separate activities. Josh, the centre manager advised Toby's parents that there was no need to separate them in daily activities, and that they were choosing to work together in the same group, so it would not be appropriate to separate them. However, Toby's parents told Josh that they would have to consider moving Toby from the centre as they did not think it was appropriate to encourage a relationship with Mandy. Josh pointed out that this had not been the case, that the two young people liked each other from the beginning and were choosing to spend time together in the social activities. Josh also advised them that they needed to speak with Toby about their intentions. After six weeks of attending the centre, Toby informed his parents that he and Mandy would like to get a flat of their own to live together.

Shortly after this Toby was admitted to hospital after having an accident at the centre where he fractured his left arm. He needed an operation to re-set the fracture and was kept in for a week for observations and monitoring. Mandy visited Toby daily while he was an inpatient, and wanted to help in Toby's care, however, she was told that this was not appropriate, as his parents had said they would assist him. Toby, however, wanted Mandy to help him and did not want to wait for his parents to visit.

Following his discharge from the orthopaedic ward, his parents wanted to keep him at home rather than send him to the centre. However, Toby insisted he wanted to go back so he could get to see Mandy. Josh advised that Toby could attend and take part in moderate activities that would not impact on the healing of his fracture. Josh contacted Toby's GP to discuss the case and to ask for a social services referral for a key worker. Toby informed his parents again one day after returning from the centre that he and Mandy wanted to find a flat of their own and move in together.

Activity 10.3   Communication

1. What are the likely reasons, if any, why Mandy was not allowed to help Toby with his care on the ward?
2. Share your views about perceptions of learning-disabled people who choose to date, have sex, get married or live with their partners.
3. What actions can be taken to support Toby and Mandy in their wish to set up home together?
4. How can the above frameworks apply here?

There is an outline answer to these questions at the end of the chapter.

It is everyone's responsibility to ensure that LD people are supported in their decision-making about their lives and making their voices heard (Chapman et al., 2024). Your contribution to this is important. Becoming a disability champion in the clinical workplace is one way of showing commitment to improving inclusivity

Supporting and enabling independent living with challenging behaviours

You are expected to have a sound understanding of appropriate ways to support those who live with an LD, whenever they are present in the care system or in any environment. Adopting an approach that is supportive and enabling is a key requirement, underpinned by person-centred care. The next scenario gives you an opportunity to consider ways that this can be possible in situations where challenging behaviours are manifested.

Scenario: Jamie

Jamie is 15 years old and has a severe learning disability (SLD). Although his speech is slow, he can make himself understood. His movements are very limited – he needs help to get out of bed and uses a supportive wheelchair to get around. Since reaching puberty, his behaviour has become disruptive and his parents find it difficult to manage him on their own. He has recently started to hit out at them, biting and kicking them when they try to get him up in the mornings. He has also begun to spit his food back at them when they tried to feed him. He also lashed out at Sam, his 12-year-old brother, hitting him in the face and swearing at him. His parents sought help with his care and were able to get him into the local day centre.

(Continued)

(Continued)

You are on a placement at the day centre when Jamie arrives for the first time. The manager asks you to oversee his care for the day. Jamie began to show sexualised behaviour towards you and other members of staff.

Activity 10.4   Critical thinking

1.   What will be the priorities for Jamie's care while he is attending the day centre?
2.   How will you be able to contribute to this?
3.   How will communication skills you have learned assist you in his care?

There is an outline answer to these questions at the end of the chapter.

Challenging behaviour is defined by NICE (2015) as behaviour that can be of an intensity, duration and frequency that it could threaten physical safety of the disabled person and other people around them. The behaviour can also severely limit the person's access to using ordinary community facilities or even impede their quality of life.

Types of challenging behaviours include: aggression, self-harming, disruption, such as tantrums, swearing, screaming and refusing to follow instructions. Some behaviours may also be violent, such as head banging or other self-harming actions, kicking, biting, punching, fighting and damaging property. Sexualised behaviours in public may also be observable as in this case.

Likely reasons could be, attention seeking, avoidance of a difficult task, sensory satisfaction, as a way of communication or expression, to let others know they are not well, or that they are uncomfortable.

A strengths-based approach supports the affirmation model discussed earlier, as it focuses on emphasising people's abilities and what they are capable of achieving, rather than on their deficits.

Valuing each person as an individual is a key underpinning factor here (Department of Health and Social Care, 2010). The aim is to recognise individuals' strengths, determination and resilience often found in families who are capable of not only learning but of growth and change, with the right support and attitude (SCIE, 2022c). Steps to promoting a strengths-based approach include valuing individuals' skills, connections, potential and knowledge (Gottlieb, 2012).

Chapter summary

This chapter explored communication practice and experiences for people living with learning disability and considered strategies for effective and interactive interventions that promote positive behaviour outcomes and living independently. You looked at the historical context, public perceptions and ways that policy and legislation have contributed to changing the narrative to one of support for those who live with a learning disability. You compared models of disability and discussed lived experiences in the context of valuing people and enabling their independence. You also considered ways of ensuring that appropriate and relevant communication strategies are used to promote positive behaviour management and change and enable clearer understanding of the needs of those who live with LD. Your responsibilities as a student nurse have been outlined. As has the importance of recognising the need to work collaboratively with other members of the interprofessional team to ensure that people who live with LD feel enabled, are supported to be independent and can achieve their own personal goals in society without fear of discrimination and marginalisation.

Activities: brief outline answers

Activity 10.1   Critical thinking (page 145)

- There are a number of factors that must be taken into account in Carmen's care. All staff should have an understanding of Down's syndrome and how it may affect individual patients (Brady et al., 2023, Clemency, 2021). Perhaps because this is a medical ward that treats diabetic patients only, members of staff may not have the skills required to work with patients who have a learning disability. There could be assumptions being made that are not evidence based, that patients who live with Down's syndrome are unable to care for themselves, be gainfully employed or can have relationships outside of their immediate families (Farrugia, 2019). All staff should update themselves on this condition so that they are aware of how Carmen can be appropriately supported. She has a key worker, Jonathan, who will be well known to her and her family and should be consulted prior to any decisions. Working with other members of the MDT is an important requirement in all cases, but specifically where patients on a unit may be considered vulnerable. Jonathan is likely to be someone who has been trained in specialist LD nursing skills, and understands Carmen's specific needs as he regularly supports her. He should be consulted and included in any decision-making relating to all aspects of her care.
- Your immediate responsibilities will be to ensure that Carmen's concerns are listened to in a sensitive manner. Prior to going to talk with her, you should familiarise yourself with her records, with your supervisor's permission, so you have an idea of what has happened so far. An assessment and care planning regime should be available to help you with this. An awareness of the Equality Act (2010), that has LD as a protected characteristic, is important to ensure that patients who live with any LD condition are treated with respect and always included in decisions about their care on all wards.

Activity 10.2   Decision-making (page 147)

- Facilities for patients who live with LD are likely to be available in mainstream hospital units on an ad hoc basis. For example, your surgical ward may be able to make adjustments such as special beds or other equipment to enable Jimmy to move around confidently. But these adjustments needed to be made before he arrived. Make sure you consider how your list compares with your peers in various other wards and regions.

- Every service provider has a responsibility to make adjustments that can facilitate appropriate care for people with LD. They should be able to meet these needs from a person-centred perspective, according to individual requirements and this can be done prior to the patient being admitted. It should not be seen as an unrealistic expectation, as policy requirements are quite clear on this matter.
- A systematic assessment of this patient's needs will have taken place; make sure you peruse this. Talk to the practitioner who performed the assessment to get background details. Communication needs to be individualised to the patient's requirements. It should be sensitive and have a therapeutic emphasis (Fleming et al., 2023). Listening skills are important here and non-verbal communication skills will ensure that the patient feels that their story is being heard (Ledger et al., 2022). You will also need to be able to communicate with the MDT and with the voluntary sector and other community organisations to be able to source support and information that will contribute to enhancing the patient's care while they are on your ward.
- The Equality Act (2010) is clear about the responsibilities of service providers to people who live with LD. Appropriate assessment should assist with ensuring that their needs are met, regardless of the level or type of disability. The Health and Social Care Act (Legislation.gov. uk, 2022) also seeks to ensure that patients are supported with a range of services from the MDT. The Mental Capacity Act (2005) supports people with LD. Take some time to explore these policies to familiarise yourself with their requirements. Given research evidence that clinical nurses don't always feel prepared to care for disabled patients (Lewis et al., 2017), you could prepare a brief for your ward team at their next meeting to update all staff about LD and gain evidence for your student portfolio.

Activity 10.3   Communication (page 151)

- Toby's parents are obviously very protective of him and may not be happy with him having a girlfriend. Staff on the ward may have their own enduring perceptions of disabled people in a relationship and may also not be happy with leaving them alone together in the room. These reasons likely feed into long-standing perceptions about people who live with LD and questions about their ability to form relationships. These all need to be examined by all concerned. Views about people who live with an LD wishing to date, live together or marry have evolved over the years. What are your thoughts on this matter?
- Based on the Equality Act (2010) Toby and Mandy should be fully supported to make their own decisions about their lives. One way of starting this process is to call a meeting of the MDT and ensure that Mandy, Toby, their parents, all key workers and those providing care meet to discuss a way forward to ensure that they are enabled in their choices.
- A focus on the social, resistance and affirmation models recognise the rights of this couple to have their needs acknowledged and met by all who care for them. The medical model approach considers them to have an impairment and so not able to form stable relationships.

Activity 10.4   Critical thinking (page 152)

- Jamie's assessment should include adopting strategies that are aimed at promoting positive behaviour changes.
- Recognise and focus on his strengths and identify what may be triggering his unwanted behaviours (Devlin et al., 2011).
- Ensure that he has consistency in his daily activities.
- Set goals and ensure that a full assessment is made that will include a behaviour intervention plan and ongoing monitoring (Challenging Behaviour Foundation, CBF, 2022).
- You will need the support of your supervisor and the team to ensure that there is a consistent approach to his care.
- Communication skills needed here include a calm approach, and an emphasis on likely reasons for behaviour.

Further reading

Adams, D, Carr, C, Marsden, D and Senior, K (2023) An Update on Informed Consent and the Effect on the Clinical Practice of Those Working with People with a Learning Disability. *Learning Disability Practice*, 26 (4).

Discusses the issues relating to informed consent relevant to practitioners who work with people who are learning disabled.

Green, J, Leadbitter, K, Ainsworth, J and Bucci, S (2022) An Integrated Early Care Pathway for Autism. *The Lancet: Child & Adolescent Health*, 6 (5): 335–344.

Explores care pathway for children and young people who live with autism.

Iqtadar, S, Hern, DI and Ellison, S (2020) If It Wasn't My Race, It Was Other Things Like Being a Woman, or My Disability: A Qualitative Research Synthesis of Disability Research. *Disability Studies Quarterly*, 40 (2).

Research paper exploring intersectional aspects of disability experiences.

MENCAP (2023) Death by Indifference: Reports on Institutional Discrimination in the NHS and the Impact of this Specifically on People Who Live with a Learning Disability. Available at: www.mencap.org.uk/sites/default/files/2016-07/DBIreport.pdf (Accessed 2 October 2023).

This report highlights the experiences of disabled service users in the NHS and presents case study examples of patients who lost their lives as a result of inadequate care.

Stefánsdóttir, S, Sigurjónsdóttir, HB and Rice, J (2023) Weapons and Tactics: A Story of Parents with Learning Disabilities Maintaining Family Integrity. *British Journal of Learning Disabilities*, 51 (1): 62–69.

Considers how parents who live with a learning disability navigate their daily lives to sustain and maintain family values and integrity.

The Guardian (2012) The Thalidomide Scandal: 60-Year Timeline. Available at www.theguardian.com/society/2012/sep/01/thalidomide-scandal-timeline (Accessed 30 August 2023).

This article gives a timeline overview of the historic issues which resulted in the use of the thalidomide drug during early pregnancy, causing disability in many children during the 1960s.

Useful websites

www.challengingbehaviour.org.uk/information-and-guidance/

Provides guidance, information, help and resources to assist families and carers with coping with challenging behaviours.

focusondisability.co.uk/

A comprehensive guide for people who live with a disability and includes details of relevant information and products to support independent living.

www.fmg.scot.nhs.uk/your-care/disability/disability-information-scotland/

Provides support and guidance to people living with a disability, their carers, families, friends and professionals who work with them.

hduhb.nhs.wales/healthcare/services-and-teams/learning-disabilities-service/

Provides specialist healthcare to adults with a diagnosed learning disability.

www.nidirect.gov.uk/information-and-services/people-disabilities

Supports people living with a disability in Northern Ireland

www.england.nhs.uk/learning-disabilities/

Discusses support for those living with a disability in England, including autism.

www.scie.org.uk/mca/introduction/mental-capacity-act-2005-at-a-glance

Provides SCIE perspectives on The Mental Capacity Act (MCA) 2005.

Chapter 11

Death, dying and bereavement: communication perspectives

Naomi Anna Watson

NMC Future Nurse: Standards of Proficiency for Registered Nurses

The following platforms and proficiencies will be covered in this chapter:

Platform 1: Being an accountable professional

1.5   Understand the demands of professional practice and demonstrate how to recognise signs of vulnerability in themselves or their colleagues and the actions required to minimise risks to health.

1.10 Demonstrate the skills and abilities required to develop, manage and maintain appropriate relationships with people, their families, carers and colleagues.

Platform 3: Provide and monitor care

3.13 Demonstrate an understanding of how to deliver sensitive and compassionate end-of-life care to support people to plan for their end of life, giving information and support to people who are dying, their families and the bereaved. Providing care to the deceased.

Platform 7: Coordinating care

7.1   Understand and apply the principles of partnership, collaboration, and interagency working across all relevant sectors.

Annexe A: Communication and relationship management skills

2.9   Engage in difficult conversations with support from others, helping people who are feeling emotionally or physically vulnerable or in distress, conveying compassion and sensitivity.

Please be aware that the case studies and scenarios detailed in this chapter contain potentially upsetting information for some readers. Please seek support from your university, tutor or supervisor if you are affected by any of the chapter content.

Introduction

Dealing with death, dying and bereavement is a life event that everyone inevitably has to face. As a nursing student or a qualified practitioner, you will no doubt come across death in your practice on a regular basis. The type and circumstances of death will vary and your contact with patients who have lost a family member will require you to understand their suffering and support them appropriately.

In this chapter, you will get the opportunity to address the impact of death, dying and bereavement on the people you care for, and explore, in the context of the available literature, how you may contribute to helping them cope with their loss, or impending loss. You also consider the types of communication skills that may be necessary while caring for people who are dying, and their families and carers who grieve.

Unexpected death

Case study: Hakeem

Hakeem was the third son of Balbir and Balvinder Kaur. He was 25 years old and in his final year at university, where he studied computer science. He frequently returned home to visit his parents. His two older brothers and one sister had completed their degrees and had taken jobs quite close to their parent's home. His family are Sikh. They met as a family at holiday times.

Hakeem had one more semester to finish his degree and was planning to stay in London after his graduation, where he intended to get a job in the city. He left his parent's home after a holiday get-together and was heading back to his university flat, but never made it.

His parents received a visit from the police that evening, to notify them that he had been in a serious road traffic accident (RTA) while driving back to university and had been admitted to an intensive care unit (ICU).

He was unconscious and had suffered injuries to his head. Hakeem's parents immediately called their other three children and they all hurried to the hospital where he had been admitted. ICU nurses and doctors advised his parents and siblings that his situation was serious. Unfortunately, within a few hours of his parents arriving in ICU, Hakeem's condition deteriorated, and he passed away that evening.

His family and friends were devastated.

Activity 11.1   Critical thinking

- Thinking about Hakeem's situation, and the impact of his accident and subsequent death on his parents and family, explain how the family could best be supported culturally, physically and emotionally, by the nurses who cared for Hakeem following his admission to ICU.
- Imagine your supervisor is one of the nurses caring for Hakeem and you were on duty with them on the day that he died. What personal support would you, as a student nurse, need and expect from them?
- Take some time to investigate what services may be available in your trust to support families from a cultural and religious perspective. For example, find out if a spiritual leader from the Sikh faith is available and could be contacted to support this family.

There is an outline answer to these questions at the end of the chapter.

According to ONS (2022a), there were 667,479 deaths in the UK in 2021, compared with 689,629, in 2020. This was the highest total number of deaths recorded since 1918, when there were 715,000. Causes of death vary between unexpected and expected deaths, however, the impact of loss will always be difficult, regardless of the circumstances and even when death is expected.

Unexpected deaths may include, but are not limited to the following examples:

- A major unexpected pandemic such as Covid-19 in 2020 (WHO, 2020b);
- RTAs such as that suffered by Hakeem, or accidents caused by an incident in the home;

- Sudden onset illnesses such as a heart attack or myocardial infarction (MI), cerebrovascular accidents (CVAs);
- Death from train and airplane crashes;
- Death from murder or suicide.

The number of people who died or were very seriously injured as a result of an RTA in the UK averaged approximately 1,560 people in 2020–21 (Department for Transport, 2023). The statistics do report that there appears to be a slight fall in the numbers, which may have been a result of the Covid-19 pandemic lockdown of 2020, during which time traffic on the roads reduced considerably as many people were forced to stay at home. None the less, it is still seen as a major cause of death in the UK and tends to fluctuate depending on the time of year. For example, there is usually an increase around Christmas time, and for many years the police have conducted annual campaigns to reduce the number of people who consume alcohol before driving. Similarly, campaigns have been launched to also reduce the numbers of people who use a mobile phone while driving, and some are still running today. In Hakeem's case, his family were told that his accident was caused by a driver who was on their mobile phone while on the motorway, crashing into his car as a result.

The death of a family member in a road traffic accident is tragic for everyone. Hakeem's parents, siblings and family were visibly very upset and openly crying. Any communication with a grieving family must take into consideration the cultural and social sensitivities of the dilemma and care must be taken to manage this with tact and compassion and awareness. To meet the needs of everyone individually and especially culturally diverse groups it is important to find out from families what their wishes are. This will mean asking direct questions relating to, for example, which spiritual leaders, if any, they wish to be called. No assumptions should ever be made as cultural or even religious groups are very rarely if ever homogenous (Watson, 2019). For this Sikh family, it is good practice that professional staff should hear directly from them specifically what kind of cultural and spiritual support they require. Therapeutic communication, when working with bereaved families, involves being able to draw on a number of tools to support them physically, emotionally and spiritually. This is just as relevant to patients as it is to their carers. Professional carers have to remain objective and calm even though they may also be deeply affected by the loss themselves.

Sharma and Gupta (2022) suggest that the value of therapeutic communication cannot be understated since it has the potential to positively impact on the experience of both the patient, where this applies, and their carers, especially those who grieve. There is, however, evidence, which suggests that nurses and healthcare professionals struggle with finding the appropriate words to say when communicating with families and carers who have suffered such a tragic loss (Patel, 2018).

Active listening skills include being able to not only give your full attention to the patient without distraction, but to also show that you are actually hearing them by providing verbal and non-verbal feedback and deferring any judgement of their presenting situation (Doyle, 2022). As part of the therapeutic communication process, this is an important professional skill to draw on when supporting distraught family members, following the unexpected death of a loved one (Underman Boggs, 2022).

Expected death: cancer

It is estimated that at least one in two people will experience cancer or will know someone who has the illness. It can affect individuals at any age. It is known that a cancer diagnosis can be very frightening, since many people are conscious that most cancers signal impending death. This is because there is as yet no cure for many types of cancers. Research is ongoing as scientists work tirelessly to find a cure for all cancers.

Breast cancer

Scenario: Sandra (Part 1)

You are on duty in a ward with your supervisor who has stepped out to the nurses' station to speak to a patient's relative. You are left alone with Sandra, a 43-year-old mother of three, who had a cancer diagnosis of the left breast three years ago. She had a mastectomy with breast reconstruction and was doing well. She began getting tingling pains in her spine and came back in for further tests. She was told by the doctors that the cancer has spread, and she has secondaries in her spine. She was admitted that morning to begin a course of chemotherapy and radiotherapy. Sandra put her head in her hands and began to sob. After a brief moment, she paused and quietly said that she was fine with her diagnosis but how worried she was for her three kids who are still only young teenagers.

Activity 11.2   Decision-making

- As a student nurse, alone in Sandra's cubicle with her, how would you respond immediately?
- What communication skills would you draw on to care for Sandra in that moment?
- At what point would you inform your supervisor of Sandra's episode of crying and about her concerns that she shared with you, for her children?

There is an outline answer to these questions at the end of the chapter.

Breast cancer mainly affects women, and it a major cause of death from cancer among women worldwide (WHO, 2020a) – it is reported that one in four women will have encountered this disease. Some men may also experience this illness, although in significantly fewer numbers.

Cancer of the breast usually begins with the detection of a lump felt by the patient, usually in one breast. On X-ray, this will show up as a lump. It has the potential to be quickly spread to other parts of the body through the lymph nodes and blood vessels, hence the importance of early detection and treatment.

In the UK, charity organisations such as Breast Cancer Now (2021) provide support for women through fundraising and leading research into breast cancer. The pink ribbon that is worn by supporters during breast cancer awareness month helps to maximise awareness of the illness and its devastating effects on patients.

In order to deal with a breast cancer diagnosis, patients need professional and family support. They will have many questions that need answering. Women who have a mastectomy may also experience feelings of loss of a body part. Even if a reconstruction has taken place, the loss can be quite acute and can bring many issues, for example understanding and managing issues of intimacy and sexuality with their partners. The impact on their mental health must be recognised and addressed. Professionals can facilitate the process of discussion by enabling women to have meaningful conversations with their partners, especially where some women may have chosen not to have breast reconstruction.

For many people, the treatment for breast cancer is initially successful, and some patients may recover fully, especially if they had an early diagnosis. Early diagnosis and treatment are important in reducing mortality rates among breast cancer patients. However, the risk of the recurrence of secondaries, also referred to as metastases in other parts of the body, as in Sandra's case, is something that patients must come to terms with and will need support and help with managing in the long term.

The World Health Organization (WHO, 2020a) reports that the burden of deaths from breast cancer is heavy in those parts of the world that are under-resourced, while death rates from the illness are steadily improving in wealthier nations. Collaborating with other nations that are experiencing reduced death rates from breast cancer is one of the ways that the WHO hopes to access resources to help under-resourced nations.

Other types of cancer

Deaths from cancer in the UK rose from 165,267 in 2017 to 166,502 in 2019 (World Cancer Research Fund, 2020). New cases diagnosed in 2019, prioritised from the highest incidence (1) to the lowest, including survival rates, are also listed below (Table 11.1)

Table 11.1 Types of cancers, new cases and survival rates in the UK, 2019 (World Cancer Research Fund, 2020).

Position (highest)	Type Of Cancer and Number of New Cases	% Mortality, 1 year	% Mortality, 5 years
1	Breast (56,987)	96.1	85.9
2	Prostate cancer (58,068)	97.2	87.9
3	Lung cancer (48,754)	43.8	19.3
4	Bowel cancer (44,706)	78.6	58.9
5	Skin cancers (17,845)		
6	Non-Hodgkins Lymphoma (13,979)		
7	Head and neck (13,049)		
8	Kidney (12,050)		
9	Pancreas (11,031)		
10	Bladder (10,515)		
11	Uterus (10,021)	89.5	75.4
12	Leukaemia (9,774)		
13	Oesophagus (92,96)		
14	Myeloma (7,138)		
15	Ovary (6,969)		

Note: No information available for blank cells. As stated earlier, the cancer burden globally continues to rise, and in the UK the problem continues to be a major cause of death. Cancer treatments also draw heavily on the use of NHS resources. Of the 387,820 total UK cancer cases diagnosed in 2019, 187,434 were among women and 200,386 were men. Numbers are predicted to continue increasing unless specific steps are taken to not only raise awareness but to encourage everyone to consider their individual lifestyle and behavioural factors that may be contributing to an increased risk of a cancer diagnosis. Recent research has identified that tackling the problem of increasing cancer rates has to recognise that improving lifestyle and behaviours such as a diet with more fruit and vegetables, physical activity, reduced smoking and a reduction in alcohol consumption must be among the targeted goals that should be considered (GBD 2019 Cancer Risk Factors Collaborators, 2022).

Scenario: Sandra (Part 2)

While you were caring for Sandra, from the case study above, she confides in you that she is very embarrassed about losing all her hair and so much body weight from her chemotherapy and radiotherapy treatment. She tells you that she does not know where to start to try and sort out the problem as she does not feel motivated. She also said she feels constantly tired and unable keep down anything she eats.

Activity 11.3 Decision-making

- How would you respond to Sandra?
- What could you do to help her with the problems that she has raised with you?

There is an outline answer to these questions at the end of the chapter.

As a student nurse, you are in an ideal position to not only listen to Sandra, but to help her think about ways she could manage the side effects of her cancer treatment. However, it is important to remember that you are not alone, and if you are unsure of how to respond, you can talk to your supervisor to get further support. For example, this could provide you with an opportunity to find out more about altered body image for female adult cancer patients, and how they may be supported to handle this problem.

Case study: Jeremy Williams

Jeremy Williams is 58 years old. His wife Hannah is 49 years old, and they have two adult children, ages 19 and 21. They have started university but have been coming back home regularly to see the family. Jeremy was diagnosed with bowel cancer, which has resulted in him having surgical resection of part of his colon. He has been left with a colostomy, an opening of the colon on his abdomen. He is still on the ward receiving post-surgery care and has become angry and upset about the outcomes of his illness. He is withdrawn and is not communicating with his wife or adult children, refusing to speak to them when they visit, or snapping at them.. Even though he has been trained by the ward staff to manage and care for his colostomy, Jeremy does not want to discuss his feelings with the staff or his family. Hannah has complained to the staff that Jeremy has become difficult, resentful and is taking out his frustration on her and the family. She is concerned because their adult children have said they won't come back to see them if he behaves the same way after discharge. She also said that if he does not want to talk about the problem, she is unsure how long she will be able to put up with his behaviour. Jeremy is due to be discharged home in a week's time.

Activity 11.4 Communication

- What specific aspects of therapeutic communication would staff require to support Jeremy?
- What available hospital and community services could nursing staff arrange to help him deal with his anger?
- How could they support Hannah, his wife?
- Find out if there is a bowel cancer support network in your trust and how referrals are made to it.

There is an outline answer to these questions at the end of the chapter.

We have previously discussed the benefits of therapeutic communication and its potential to ensure that patients feel listened to and heard when they are struggling with physical changes that they have to accept as a result of their illness, or with bereavement. Having to cope with a colostomy is a major physical change for Jeremy, and also for his wife. They will need early and continuing support to manage this phase of their lives, especially after discharge. As a student, you will also need the support of your placement supervisor to help you with caring for this family. A local support network consisting of others who may have gone through a similar issue could provide one solution to helping the family come to terms with the issue. As Jeremy's wife has already told you and your supervisor that she is concerned about his current attitude, getting the couple support from psychological services will be an important aspect of the early agenda for their care before he is discharged home.

Case study: Angie

Fiona is a third year nursing student who has been making home visits along with her supervisor Amina to Angie Green, a 42-year-old multiple sclerosis patient. Angie is a mother of two and was diagnosed at 32 years old.

In the past two years, she has begun to deteriorate to the extent that she needs 24-hour care and can only go out in a wheelchair. Her husband Jason is her main carer. Angie is now unable to speak without aid, and has difficulty swallowing, so has to be fed by a nasogastric tube. On Fiona and Amina's last visit to their home, Angie and Jason informed them that Angie wished to end her life, and that they have begun to explore the options.

Activity 11.5   Critical thinking

- In what specific ways could Amina and Fiona support this family?
- What theories could they draw on to help them?
- Find out and make a list of which countries currently legally allow assisted death by euthanasia, and how it works.
- Share your thoughts with your peers about the communication skills that you and your clinical supervisor would need to draw on in this sort of case.

There is an outline answer to these questions at the end of the chapter.

The main issue for carers, families and professional carers is how to support the patient and family to enable a good quality of life.

Euthanasia is not legal in the UK, so it is important to have up-to-date information about legal processes in order to support patients like Angie. The case of Diane Pretty is a well-known example of a patient who went to the European Court of Human Rights to gain the legal right to end her life. Her arguments were based on her conviction that the right to life also included her right to decide whether or not she wished to stay alive. However, the court did not agree with her, and she eventually died on 11 May 2002, aged just 43 years old. Diane was diagnosed with motor neurone disease in 1999. Although she would have had treatment to help alleviate her illness, her death was from complications from her condition, including respiratory problems affecting her lungs. Diane died less than three years after her diagnosis. You may also be aware of Stephen Hawking, the well-known British scientist who lived with motor neurone disease for 55 years following his diagnosis.

Palliative care: principles and practices

Scenario: Sandra (Part 3)

Sandra has deteriorated and is unable to walk. She needs 24-hour support and care. On a visit to her home with your clinical supervisor, Sandra informs you both that she would like to stay at home but is very conscious of the tremendous strain this is having on her husband and children. She is complaining of severe intermittent pain, which is becoming worse daily. She requests to be transferred to a local hospice but had to be placed on a waiting list as there were no beds available when she requested it.

Your supervisor requested the services of the Macmillan nurse to support Sandra at home while she waited for a place in the local hospice.

Activity 11.6   Team working

- Find out about the role of the Macmillan nurse in the support of terminally ill patients.
- What else could you and your supervisor do to support Sandra?
- What could you do to support Sandra's husband and teenage children at this difficult time?
- Identify the assessment processes, including pain assessment, that were used to plan appropriate care for Sandra and find out if this differs in other trusts by asking your peers.
- Talk to your student peers and find out if availability of palliative services are the same in their region/trust. For example, do hospices have a waiting list in other regions/trusts?

There is an outline answer to these questions at the end of the chapter.

Palliative care relieves patients' symptoms and prevents undue suffering, thereby enabling patients to have an acceptable quality of life during their final stages of living. This care will differ depending on the stages of the illness of an individual. For example, someone who is undergoing the terminal stages of their disease may require different support to a patient who is at the very beginning of their diagnosis (NICE, 2019).

Theories of dying, bereavement and grief work

The care of families following the death of a patient is an important aspect of required support for grief. In the case of expected death, grief and grief work will be influenced by a range of issues relating to length of, and type of illness. Borgstrom and Pearce (2022) argue that death is a social process and cannot be restricted by timed frameworks or stages of grieving. Grief work can therefore start before death and this needs to be recognised by those providing care and support to patients and their families.

In some cultures, most expected deaths are likely to happen either in hospitals, hospices, or nursing homes. Consequently, some people are reluctant to talk about, discuss, or face up to death and dying. Thanatology, which is the scientific study of death, was originally influenced by the need to raise and keep an awareness of death and dying as dying was withdrawn from the home to hospitals, hospices and nursing homes. The death awareness movement, which started in the 1950s in both the US and the UK was a major influence on the introduction of this field of study (Foseca and Testoni, 2012). The exploration of the ethical, physical, psychological, social, spiritual and cultural aspects of death and dying through the study of thanatology aims to provide a basis for reflective and constructive thinking. This is within a discipline where those wishing to do so can contribute to building up a theory base. As a student nurse, you will come across many opportunities to support families through various stages of their experiences, so an understanding of the theoretical processes will be a useful background.

Scenario: Sandra (Part 4)

Sandra was eventually able to get a place in a local hospice for her end-of-life care following metastases from breast cancer that spread to her spine. This was her personal choice. In the hospice she was supported by specialist Macmillan nurses. Her husband and children were able to visit and stay with her. She required 24-hour support and felt much more comfortable being in an environment where there were other people around her and continuous availability of staff. She sadly died six weeks after being admitted to the

(Continued)

(Continued)

hospice. Despite her expected death, her husband and children were devastated. Eleven--year-old Ginny's behaviour deteriorated following Sandra's admission to the hospice, but her behaviour became worse following her mum's death. She started playing truant from school, and her dad noticed cut marks on her wrists. She failed her end-of-year exams and started to socialise with people her dad was not happy with. He admitted that he did not know how to cope.

Activity 11.7   Reflection

- Thinking about this family's situation, in what specific ways could Sandra's widower be supported through this crisis?
- How could the children, Ginny in particular, be supported?
- Reflect on the impact Sandra's death might have on you and your supervisor. What support services are available to you as professional carers?

There is an outline answer to these questions at the end of the chapter.

Theories of dying, grief and bereavement help to identify the processes that individuals go through to try and deal with dying or losing someone. Most theorists attempt to provide a systematic process through which people grieve, however, they do not all agree with each other. Current contemporary theorists consider the concept of a staged process to be simplistic and failing to fully grasp the issues facing those who grieve (Corr, 2018, Borgstrom and Pearce, 2022). Kubler-Ross's (1969) five stages of grief is a well-known example, which identifies a staged process of dealing with the death of someone close. Kubler-Ross named the five stages as:

- anger;
- denial;
- depression/guilt;
- bargaining;
- acceptance.

The general agreement is that individuals must be allowed their rite of passage through each stage to enable their recovery. It is acknowledged, however, that these stages may not happen in the order suggested by Kubler-Ross, and the timings are also flexible, with some individuals perhaps taking longer to work through these stages. Parkes (1972), another bereavement stage theorist, suggests four stages (see Figure 11.1).

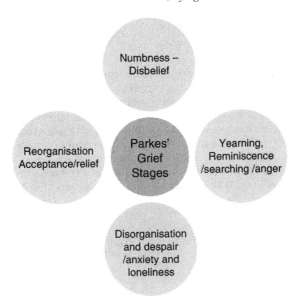

Figure 11.1   Parkes' four stages of grief (1972)

Parkes considers these stages to be part of a dynamic process that may also vary without specific timings as this will depend on the individual. Opposing authors argue that these stages fail to take into account individuals' personal inner characteristics (Corr, 2018). The dual process model of coping with grief, on the other hand, suggests that an individual's own locus of control, such as notions of resilience, come into play as families try to make sense of death and their grief (Schut, 1999, Gorman, 2011).

Chapter summary

In this chapter you looked at death, dying and bereavement and the issues that affect patients, their carers and families. You considered these from the context of expected and unexpected deaths, including euthanasia and assisted dying and their demographical profiles. You considered the impact of dying and bereavement on patients, carers and families. You looked at thanatology and other theories of death, dying and bereavement when considering the impact on families. You also looked at support systems that are available to promote your mental health and wellbeing and that of your supervisor.

Communicating with patients, carers and their families during difficult life experiences such as actual or impending death, whether expected or unexpected, can be challenging for everyone. As a learner you have the opportunity to develop professional communication skills in clinical practice. These will enable you to better support those you care for, whether it is with breaking bad news or helping individuals, carers and families deal with difficult aspects of their situation.

Activities: brief outline answers

Activity 11.1   Critical thinking (page 159)

When Hakeem was still alive and unconscious, nurses and medical staff would have spent time with the family explaining his brain damage injuries and any likelihood, if any, of recovery. Nursing support would include ensuring that the family are able to talk through their distress, so listening skills will be an essential aspect of care. They will also require the space to grieve in whatever way they desire. In some cultures, some men may not grieve openly, and consider their role as being strong in order to support their partner and other members of the family. In other cultures, however, it may be normal for everyone to openly cry as they grieve and mourn following the death of close family members. Reactions of the family may therefore vary, even from generational perspectives. It is important that nurses recognise and respond to the specific societal, cultural and religious support that that the whole family will need to help them through this difficult time.

Your reaction to the death of such a young patient could also affect you emotionally. Your clinical supervisor will be your first line of support. Your family and your peers will additionally prove to be invaluable in helping you to cope.

Your supervisor may also be very upset but again they may be familiar with these experiences working in an ICU. You may both need further help with your own wellbeing, however, so seeking out emotional support will be an important part of self-care for all staff concerned.

Activity 11.2   Decision-making (page 161)

Hopefully your immediate response would be to stay with Sandra and allow her to cry for as long as she needed to. You could then find out from her what she may need at that time, and wait for her to respond. You should actively listen and give her your full attention.

You would wait with her until your supervisor returns, at which time you could offer to make her a hot drink.

It would be best to wait until after the episode to inform your supervisor outside of the room, about Sandra's earlier distress and concerns for her children, in case this needed further exploration.

Activity 11.3   Decision-making (page 164)

Your conversation with Sandra would include finding out whether she has explored any options previously about what to do about her hair loss. You may wish to check if there are any local breast cancer support networks in the trust or in her local community that she can access for further help. You may want to find out if there are other inpatients with a similar diagnosis, and if there is any ward support that may be useful for her.

Activity 11.4   Communication (page 164)

Once again, it will be helpful to apply therapeutic communication skills to provide support for Jeremy. Active listening, appropriate non-verbal cues, reflecting back when required will all be very useful. You should be able to work with your supervisor to arrange the relevant services such as a psychologist, a social worker, or other locally available services, depending on the locality. Listening to Hannah and giving her the space to speak to a professional person in confidence will be helpful in enabling her to be heard.

Activity 11.5   Critical thinking (page 165)

You will require support from your supervisor when discussing euthanasia with Jason and Angie. Once again, therapeutic communication skills will be a vital support for you both. Hopefully you will have had an opportunity to read around the subject of assisted dying before going to see the family. If not, this is something to do following the visit. In this couple's case, Borgstrom and Pearce's (2022) theory of death as a social process may be considered, since Angie is still alive, and the couple are aware of her impending death. You can also find out the current situation regarding assisted deaths in the UK, and which countries allow this. Switzerland is a very common destination for people wishing to be assisted with dying. Patients are assisted by a medical doctor, using a lethal injection.

Activity 11.6   Team working (page 166)

The best way to find out about the role of the Macmillan nurse is to speak to one. It would be useful to set up a 15-minute appointment in conjunction with your clinical supervisor to talk to one about their role.

Both you and your supervisor can offer emotional support to Sandra, and her family, as she will be familiar with you both and will be reassured with familiar faces.

You will need to find out about available services that they can access and ensure they are referred.

Assessment tools in use within different NHS trusts are likely to vary, so it is important for you to speak to your supervisor and identify the ones being used in your setting. You can also check with your peers to see how these may differ in each trust. The National Institute for Health and Care Excellence (NICE, 2019) has provided guidelines for assessing and delivering palliative care to those who are deemed to be approaching the end of their lives.

Activity 11.7   Reflection (page 168)

As you reflect on the events with which the family has been living for a considerable time, it is useful to consider psychological support for Sandra's partner and their three children. Ginny will need to be referred to the child and adolescent family services team for appropriate support.

You and your supervisor should ensure that your own mental health and wellbeing is supported as well. Most trusts now have staff support networks that can be accessed for help. Talking therapy services can be a useful opportunity to speak with available staff counselling services to help.

Further reading

Cancer.net (2022) Understanding Grief Within a Cultural Context. Available at : www.cancer. net/coping-with-cancer/managing-emotions/grief-and-loss/understanding-grief-within-cultural-context (Accessed 15 January 2024).

Gives an overview about cultural factors that may affect dying and the grieving process.

Provides support for those who are grieving from the perspective of someone who has had a similar experience.

Useful websites

breastcancernow.org

Statistical details about breast cancer and its global impact.

www.cruse.org.uk/about/

Cruse bereavement support.

https://griefjourney.com/welcome-to-grief-journey-co-uk-the-u-k-home-of-the-centre-for-the-grief-journey

A support network available for grieving families in the UK.

www.macmillan.org.uk

Provides information about end-of-life care for individuals and families.

www.mariecurie.org.uk

Support network for families who are grieving.

www.who.int/news/item/08-03-2021-new-global-breast-cancer-initiative-highlights-renewed-commitment-to-improve-survival

Explores breast cancer initiatives across the world from a global perspective.

Chapter 12

Communication with compassion

Naomi Anna Watson

NMC Future Nurse: Standards of Proficiency for Registered Nurses

The following platforms and proficiencies will be covered in this chapter:

Platform 1: Being an accountable professional

1.17 Take responsibility for continuous self-reflection, seeking and responding to support and feedback to develop their professional knowledge and skills.

Platform 2: Promoting health and preventing ill health

2.5 Promote and improve the mental, physical, behavioural and other health-related outcomes by understanding and explaining the principles, practice and evidence base for health screening programmes.

Platform 4: Providing and evaluating care

4.3 Demonstrate the knowledge, communication and relationship and management skills required to provide people, families and carers with accurate information that meets their needs before, during and after a range of interventions.

Platform 6: Improving safety and quality of care

6.11 Acknowledge the need to accept and manage uncertainty and demonstrate an understanding of strategies that develop resilience in self and others.

Annexe A: Communication and relationship management skills

1.1 Actively listen, recognise and respond to verbal and non-verbal cues.
1.2 Use prompts and positive verbal and non-verbal reinforcement.
1.3 Use appropriate non-verbal communication, including touch, eye contact and personal space.
1.4 Make appropriate use of open and closed questioning.

(Continued)

(Continued)

1.5   Use caring conversation techniques.

1.6   Check understanding and use clarification techniques.

1.7   Be aware of unconscious bias in communication encounters.

2.3   Recognise and accommodate sensory impairments during all communications.

2.4   Support and manage the use of personal communication aids.

2.8   Provide information and explanation to people, families and carers and respond to questions about their treatment and care and possible ways of preventing ill health to enhance understanding.

Chapter aims

After reading this chapter, you will be able to:

- define compassion in the context of communication and apply this to non-English speakers;
- discuss ways of supporting and engaging compassionately in communication with peers and colleagues;
- outline the basis of the 6Cs and their importance to your practice as they relate to policy and research perspectives;
- use a model of reflection to examine your role as a student and eventual qualified practitioner in the promotion of communication that reflects compassion.

Introduction

So far in this book you have explored different aspects of communication and looked at its application in a variety of nursing and healthcare situations across the lifespan.

In this chapter you get the opportunity to focus on issues that are relevant and necessary for communication with compassion. To do this you consider a range of factors that can influence your attempts to ensure that compassion is an underpinning aspect of how you relate to people as a student nurse and eventually as a qualified practitioner. You will also explore how your communication skills for effective practice can be improved and strengthened and be able to apply policy and research perspectives to your communication patterns. You reflect on your role as an emerging qualified practitioner in promoting communication skills in practice that embody compassion, not just to patients, but to their carers, families and to your peers and colleagues.

Defining compassion

Being able to communicate with compassion is a learned skill that must be supported by sound evidence-based knowledge to underpin its manifestation in practice. It cannot be assumed that compassionate communication is simply possible without active preparation prior to being faced with situations in the clinical environment that require sensitivity, kindness and empathy. We know this because of numerous examples of a lack of care and compassion being provided in practice in the NHS. The Francis Report (Francis, 2013), is one such example where following a public enquiry into the Mid-Staffordshire NHS Foundation Trust, the conclusions were that the important fundamental principles of safety and responsibility in the provision of care for patients were compromised, resulting in harm to many patients. This report specifically cited a lack of effective communication between patients and healthcare professionals as a major failure in care delivery practice. The knowledge gained from exploring the variety of topics in this book provides a sound background that can be used to practice compassionate communication. For example, in an earlier chapter of this book (see Chapter 1) you had the opportunity to practise with your peers the very basic skill of always ensuring that you introduce yourself to patients, their carers, families and clients as far as this is possible. This simple act is sometimes ignored in clinical practice, according to the evidence base (Grainger, 2013) and very soon becomes embedded, adopted by everyone, to the detriment of patient care. Introducing yourself to colleagues, patients and others in the workplace has the potential to be of immense value especially to anxious patients, their carers and families who desperately need reassurance and information about their illness. To communicate with compassion is to be able to actively and intentionally address basic, taken-for-granted, communication skills while remaining conscious of the needs of the other person, especially those who may be suffering and are anxious about their illness (Reid et al., 2016). At the heart of this intentionality is respect for the other person, and an active resolve to treat them with dignity and compassion (Su et al., 2020). This is the underpinning basis of 'person-centred care' (Kerr et al., 2022).

Being able to interact from the position of understanding the needs of patients and being willing to relate to them with kindness must involve deliberate engagement with them through listening skills, while recognising and affirming their individual verbal and non-verbal cues. The case study that follows provides an example by focusing on a case that encourages you to think about compassionate communication with someone whose first language is not English.

Case study: Khalid

Khalid is a young male refugee who appears to be around 25 years old. He was admitted to A&E following a severe asthma attack. His first language is Arabic, and he speaks a little English, using only single word responses. On admission he appears to be able to understand

(Continued)

(Continued)

more than he is able to speak. Staff became aware of this because they noted that he could follow basic commands, such as 'raise your right hand', 'what is your name', 'how old are you'. They therefore assumed that he could speak English. On arrival he was distressed and wheezing heavily, with severe shortness of breath and coughing excessively. When asked how long he had suffered with asthma and if he had been treated before, he responded in his first language, and no one was able to understand what he was saying. His breathlessness also made it very difficult for him to speak and he was catching his breath while trying to express himself, becoming more and more distressed with each attempt. The charge nurse, Matthew, kept telling him to speak in English as he had already responded to other basic questions. He tried to respond but again in Arabic, and with no coherence to his speech. Matthew again insisted that he speaks in English and reminded him that they knew he could speak English. He became frustrated and began to shout, panic and become very restless, which made his condition worse. Khalid needed urgent emergency care to improve his breathlessness and reduce his anxiety, while also starting treatment for his asthma. As this was his first time in that hospital, there were no previous records and admissions staff were unable to get a full history from him when he first arrived, or to ascertain if he had been admitted anywhere else before. After many unsuccessful attempts at getting a full history for an initial assessment, the A&E team eventually proceeded to treat Khalid to relieve his breathlessness and attempt to stabilise his condition.

Activity 12.1   Decision-making

1.   What would you say are the priorities required for Khalid's care?
2.   How could compassionate communication be applied in this case?
3.   How could his initial assessment be better managed?

There is an outline answer to these questions at the end of the chapter.

There are many factors that may present as barriers to caring effectively and compassionately for Khalid. Cultural challenges could limit and negatively affect communication with him (Babaei and Taleghani, 2019). Ways that race and ethnicity influence communication patterns was covered in a previous chapter (see Chapter 4). Barriers caused by language differences can compromise care outcomes unless active steps are taken to reduce this. The tendency to rely on family and friends for communicating with those whose first language is not English is a fairly common practice. In Khalid's case, there were no relatives to help. However, there are issues to be aware of if relatives or friends are available and ready to help in your care environment. For example, using children as interpreters for their parents does not guarantee accuracy of the required information. It will depend on the sensitivities of the subject being explored and could severely compromise confidentiality. The Equality Act (Legislation.gov.uk, 2010) requires the provision of alternative forms of communication that should use an inclusive and equitable approach. Telephone interpreting services are now widely available and provide an alternative method to using relatives and friends. At the heart of compassionate communication with those whose first language is not English is the requirement to show sensitivity and empathy to how they may be feeling. Demonstrating actions that represent basic kindness and understanding of their fears and anxiety is essential. Being able to identify any likely implicit biases that you may have will help you to limit its effect on how you treat others at work (Todt, 2023). Examples of bias include assumptions that a patient may be pretending not to be able to speak English, especially when they seem to understand you. Refugee or other patients who are distressed, anxious and unwell could revert to the use of their first language even if they speak some English. They may struggle to communicate and could also appear to show aggressive behaviour patterns that reflect their frustrations with not being able to make themselves understood.

Compassionate caring includes being cognitively aware and understanding of someone's suffering, showing concern and sympathy, wanting to relieve that person's suffering and being willing and ready to help relieve their suffering (Babaei and Taleghani, 2019). Allaying the patient's anxiety is the main priority. Therapeutic touch is widely used in clinical practice, recognised as a way of reassuring patients that professionals are committed to helping them recover (Mendes et al., 2022). Understanding the cultural implications though, is important to ensure its appropriateness in all situations.

Compassionate communication with peers and colleagues

The healthcare environment is considered to be quite a stressful one for most patients, who usually arrive anxious and worried. They may be in pain and experiencing symptoms of illnesses that they may not know much about. Their anxiety may at times make them appear aggressive (Bramley and Matiti, 2014). Members of staff who have to work in that environment may also view it as highly stressful, especially if they are new or are having to work under excessive pressure because of inadequate staffing, low resources, or other service disruptions (Cooksley et al., 2023).

The ability to respond and recognise when people are suffering or are upset and scared is a core aspect of communicating with compassion. This also applies to your peers and colleagues in education or clinical practice who require a compassionate approach to their problems. However, at times issues such as power relationships and hierarchical workplace systems and structures may interfere with the ability to show empathy and communicate compassionately (Arkan et al., 2020) (see also Chapter 2 in this book). Being a part of the multidisciplinary team (MDT) gives you many opportunities to demonstrate your learning and apply it when dealing with healthcare professionals in the workplace, including fellow nurses, whether as colleagues or learners. Chapter 5 explored MDT working in more detail. The next scenario focuses specifically on your peers and provides an illustration for you to consider.

Scenario: Leslie

Leslie is a first-year student who is new to your ward environment, where you have been placed as a third-year student three weeks prior to her arrival. The ward is a large 32-bed medical geriatric ward, with four individual rooms and you have been asked by your supervisor to support Leslie and ensure that she is orientated to the ward. This is Leslie's very first time in a large-ward environment and she is obviously very nervous. She confides in you that she lacks confidence and worries about whether she has made the right choice of career. While you were showing her around, you arrive in the room of Daphne Green, an 89-year-old lady who appeared to be taking a nap. She did not respond to your call and on checking further, you realised that she was not breathing. You are aware that Daphne is on a 'do not resuscitate' (DNR) order so you told Leslie to wait and went out to get your supervisor. Leslie was scared of being left alone and immediately ran out of the room after you. You were unhappy with her response and told her to do as she was told and stay there until you got back. Your supervisor arrived and told Leslie to go and get the doctor on call. Leslie did not know which number to call and did not realise that the doctor was already on the ward. Following the incident, you were asked to take charge of last offices for Daphne, and you and Leslie prepared to undertake this activity together before the arrival of family members to pay their last respects. As it was a busy day on the ward, you were unable to speak with Leslie to debrief her or to ask how she felt about the day's events, but without telling her, you decided that you would do so in the morning when you were both on again on the same shift. The next morning you arrive on duty to a message left by Leslie that she would not be returning to the ward, and she is thinking about withdrawing from her studies.

Activity 12.2   Leadership and management

1. In what ways could Leslie's first day on a large ward be better managed, and was it fair of your supervisor to ask you to buddy her?
2. Consider the communication skills that support you as you try to orientate her onto the ward environment.
3. What actions can you and your supervisor take to further support Leslie, going forward, given her decision to probably leave the profession?

There is an outline answer to these questions at the end of the chapter.

Buddying up with peers who are in their first or second year in clinical practice is a good way of developing and demonstrating your leadership and management potential. Good leadership at work rests significantly on how everyone is treated and ensuring that compassionate communication underpins your approach is an important requirement for leadership development in the workplace (King's Fund, 2022). Compassionate leadership includes the following aspects:

- showing awareness of other people's needs;
- having a non-judgemental approach to the viewpoints of others;
- fostering resilience and tolerance when dealing with people who are suffering personal distress;
- having the ability to demonstrate and feel empathy as required, towards everyone during all stages of professional life;
- taking responsibility and accountability as the leader, for all team outcomes, whether good or bad.

As a student nurse, you are required to utilise the opportunity to practise and develop leadership skills in the workplace. You will be expected to mentor and supervise junior students such as Leslie, in practice. It is hence important to recognise your responsibility to support others in the workplace by being kind, showing empathy and enabling a work environment where others feel they can grow and thrive (Kerr et al., 2023).

The 6Cs and their implications for nursing practice

Within nursing and healthcare, the 6Cs are essential aspects of professional practice and are considered to be major motivators driving the choice to become a healthcare professional. The introduction of the 6Cs happened as a result of reports on the failings of healthcare following incidents such as the Mid-Staffordshire scandal. The values were embedded as essential aspects of care delivery practice required to improve patient satisfaction and care quality improvement. The following case study gives you an opportunity to consider some of these skills.

Case study: Jeremy Grant

Jeremy Grant arrived on the ward from the A&E Department. He is 84 years old and suffers from dementia. Jeremy recently lost his wife Sally, who had been his main carer. They lived together until her passing, when Jeremy had to move into a nursing home. They had three children who all live and work abroad. Jeremy arrived unaccompanied from the nursing home

(Continued)

(Continued)

to have his diabetes stabilised. A message in his records said that while at the nursing home he received regular visits from Lillian, the admiral nurse. On arrival he was upset and confused. He began to shout and refused to let anyone touch him. He got off the trolley but was reluctant to get into bed. Jeremy was placed in a side room and Bethany, the nurse in charge, asked Frank the student nurse to remain with him until he became calmer. Jeremy told Frank that he needed to get back home to Sally and that he was worried that she was on her own. He also said that he had been working out of town for a few weeks and had not heard from her and was worried about her. He began to pace the floor and asked Frank if he could assist him to get home to check on Sally. Frank reminded Jeremy that his wife had passed away, and that he no longer worked but had been admitted from a nursing home. Jeremy became angry and told him he was wrong and that all he wanted was some help to get back home to Sally.

Activity 12.3   Critical thinking

Outline the ways that Frank will be able to demonstrate compassionate communication from the perspectives of the 6Cs.

There is an outline answer to this question at the end of the chapter.

The values described in the 6Cs (Figure 12.1) were introduced in order to transform nursing practice by ensuring that all patients had access to high-quality care that was dignified, respectful, compassionate and relevant to their needs. They were in response to many reports of poor care being provided across the NHS, which triggered public concern and led to a number of public inquiries, including the Francis Report (Francis, 2013).

Care: Enabling and supporting patients through a personalised approach to care delivery.

Compassion: Ensuring dignity, empathy, kindness and respect in all circumstances and acknowledging patients' needs from each individual perspective.

Competence: Having the clinical expertise and technical knowledge where it is required to ensure effective evidence-based practice interventions.

Communication: Applying active listening, verbal and non-verbal skills, accurate documentation in team working and care relationships.

Courage: Acting as an advocate where required, speaking up as appropriate, being prepared to challenge the actions of others in the workplace when required if there are concerns, doing the right thing. Having the vision and personal strength to innovate and embrace new ways of working.

Commitment: Taking action in response to a vision to improve care experiences of patients and service users.

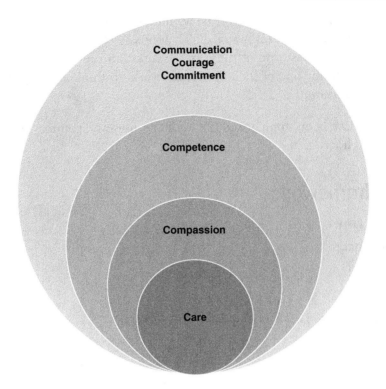

Figure 12.1 The 6Cs of nursing (RCN, 2015)

These values are essential underpinning aspects of the way you develop your practice as a healthcare professional and are just as applicable to your interaction with your peers and colleagues as your interaction with patients, their carers and families.

Reflection on compassionate communication: end-of-life perspective

By now you would have been introduced to reflection as part of your learning process as a student nurse and eventual qualified practitioner. Effective reflection is a tool that gives you an analytical insight into the way you practise and helps you think about any likely strengths, limitations or future actions that could improve and extend your learning from specific actions. There are three main ways of applying reflexivity as part of your learning:

- reflection-in-action: While engaged in a clinical event;
- reflection-on-action: Looking back at an incident;
- reflection-for-action: Considering the next steps.

(Thompson and Thompson, 2023)

A number of reflective frameworks can be applied to assist professional practitioners, (Jasper, 2013, Schon, 1987, Freshwater, 2007, Johns, 2022, Gibbs 2013). You should already be aware of at least one of these frameworks, and in this section, you get an opportunity to apply any one of the above frameworks to think about and reflect on a communication encounter.

The ones above have been summarised for you here, however, you may have found others that you can choose to use.

Reflective frameworks

- ERA cycle (Jasper, 2013)
  - Experience
  - Reflection
  - Action

- Driscoll (2007) based on Terry Borton's 1970s model
  - What
  - So what
  - Now what?

- Kolb's (1984) experiential learning model
  - Concrete experience
  - Reflective observation
  - Abstract conceptualisation
  - Active experimentation

- Gibbs' (1988) reflective cycle
  - Description
  - Feelings
  - Evaluation
  - Analysis
  - Conclusion
  - Action plan

Scenario: Amber

You are on placement in a hospice/end-of-life ward as a final year student nurse. Amber Green has been an inpatient for three weeks. She has pancreatic cancer and has been receiving palliative care. You have been caring for Amber with your supervisor. Amber has been gradually getting weaker and unable to mobilise or attend to her own activities of daily living. She complained that the pain is getting worse, and she wants to increase the dose she is having. This was restricted by the medical team to four times a day only as it was making Amber very drowsy and unable to stay awake. You and your supervisor spoke to the medical team to request that her pain medication move to on demand, so she could access this herself whenever required. Amber's carer and family approached you to ask you to restrict Amber's access to more pain relief medication as they would like to be able to spend time with her during her final days where she is conscious and aware. You assumed that she had discussed this with them and informed the doctor without talking to your supervisor. The doctor restricted the dose as requested. Amber became upset and wanted to know why her pain medication had been restricted. She told you that she did not discuss her increased pain with her family as she did not wish to upset them further. She did not want them to know that she had asked for more pain relief, and did not wish to self-medicate, just for the dose to be increased. Your supervisor advised that you should have talked to her first before engaging the doctor.

Activity 12.4   Reflection

Choose any model of reflection with which you are familiar and reflect on this incident, using the prompts provided.

As this activity is based on your own reflection, there is no outline answer.

Williams (2023) identifies challenges that professionals face when caring for those who are at the end of their life. At times communication can be misunderstood by the care team and by patients and families. How you navigate these issues requires sensitivity and an understanding of the dilemmas that patients may sometimes feel as they try to reduce any distress for their families. There are many instances when the patient may require us to make decisions for them that they have chosen not to discuss with family members. Working closely with the MDT and remembering that you do not have to make these decisions alone will help to alleviate the issues faced.

Reflecting on your role as a student nurse and on the way you communicate is a required way of strengthening and developing an awareness of your practice. It provides the potential for you to learn more about yourself and how you relate to service users and colleagues not only in clinical settings but in educational environments. You are able to strengthen your critical thinking skills and identify ways to improve your future performance in any aspect of your professional practice. Using a reflective journal helps to structure your learning from your experience so that your future actions become specific learning points that can influence your practice going forward.

Chapter summary

In this chapter you explored communication in the context of compassionate care. You were able to define compassion in the context of communication. You looked at levels of compassion and how this can be manifested in the patient experience. You outlined the basis of the 6Cs and their importance in clinical practice and considered ways that will contribute to improving and strengthening the development of communication skills for practice. You identified policy and research perspectives to your communication style in clinical practice and applied a framework to reflect on your role as an eventual qualified practitioner in the promotion of communication that reflects compassion. The results will be increased patient satisfaction and strengthening of patient/nurse relationships, an improvement in care quality and overall better likelihood for positive health outcomes. Your professional practice will also be enhanced as you apply the skills you learned when you move into your new status of qualified practitioner.

Activities: brief outline answers

Activity 12.1   Decision-making (page 176)

The priorities for Khalid's care must begin with a compassionate attitude, to include basic introductions, reassurance and attention to his anxiety by ensuring that he receives help with breathing as soon as possible, even before questioning him for history and assessment purposes. This will be to alleviate his breathing with appropriate medication and promote a calm and reassuring environment. He appears to understand some commands although he responds with one word only at a time, so therapeutic communication skills will be important in this care episode. Primarily a calm demeanour will ensure that his anxiety reduces as his breathing goes back to near normal levels. Staff will be required to demonstrate the use of any instruments that they wish to use to measure his breathing, such as the administration of oxygen to support his breathing, the use of an intravenous infusion, a peak-flow monitor or other device, including any inhalers that he will eventually need to be shown how to use. Since it is known that he understands some English, this should be helpful, however, any ongoing distress will limit his ability to follow instructions.

Compassionate communication for Khalid needs to reflect cultural sensitivity and recognition of his struggles with the English language. Arranging an online interpreter to help complete a full assessment will be the next priority once he has been stabilised. Showing an awareness of personal cultural worldview and recognising individual attitudes towards cultural competence will help with developing cross-cultural skills. An understanding of different cultures, recognising his strengths and limitations, and finding ways to enable his cooperation will assist in gaining his trust.

Once Khalid's immediate needs for safety have been met, staff can concentrate on an assessment that will provide details about his past history and any treatment he has had elsewhere.

Activity 12.2   Leadership and management (page 178)

As a student nurse in your final year of practice, you would have acquired a range of knowledge and skills to use to support a first-year student who is joining the clinical environment. A junior student brings an opportunity for you to act as a buddy to encourage and support them in practice. Your code of conduct requires you to be able and willing to support other peers in practice as a senior student and a soon-to-be qualified practitioner (NMC, 2018). You may have considered that

Leslie's first day was in the main, managed very well. One aspect of working in clinical healthcare environments is that it is difficult to predict what may happen at any given time. You were not to know that a patient in a room would have passed away, so that was an unpredictable event. A death is always a difficult and traumatising event for everyone, but especially so for someone who is new to the ward and may not have seen a dead person previously. In this scenario then, it is not easy to say what could have been done differently to better manage the situation, except to perhaps recognise Leslie's status as a learner who is just observing on the first day. So it may not have been appropriate to ask her to stay while you fetch your supervisor or for her to be asked to fetch the doctor, since she had not yet been introduced to the team and did not know who they were, except for your supervisor.

Having covered many concepts in this book, you can draw on a wide range of skills to communicate with compassion to your peers. For example, using conversation techniques that are caring could have included sharing with Leslie some experiences from your own time as a student in your first year, and what helped you to cope and strengthen your resilience. An empathic approach to her uncertainties on her first day in the clinical setting would have helped her as she navigated this new experience (Öztürk and Kaçan, 2022, Reid, et al., 2016). Using non-verbal cues by giving her a reassuring touch or hug where appropriate may have helped to allay her fears. Therapeutic touch can also be a supportive gesture to peers and colleagues who may become distressed at work (Burgess et al., 2023).

Informing her about the types of patients usually present on the ward and checking with her about her previous experiences of death and dying may also have given her the chance to share her fears.

You, your supervisor and Leslie, should have had an opportunity to meet as a threesome following the incident to talk through the events and check that Leslie was coping. She went home that day without having an opportunity to talk through her experience. The fact that she chose not to return the next day could indicate that she may have felt unsupported. This should trigger a reflective plan for you as a final year student, which you could discuss with your supervisor and consider how you both may be able to reach out to Leslie to help her to change her mind about leaving.

Activity 12.3   Critical thinking (page 180)

In caring for Jeremy, Frank has the opportunity to think creatively. Care includes providing a personalised approach, and working directly with Jeremy is a good opportunity to get to know him better.

Frank could start with introducing himself, finding out how Jeremy prefers to be addressed and beginning to establish a relationship of trust, by actively listening to Jeremy's story and asking pertinent questions in line with his responses. For example, he could ask how long Jeremy had been married, number of children and which country they now lived in (Barker and Williams, 2018). Frank should also find an opportunity to ask Jeremy about his diabetes and treatment so that this can begin as soon as possible. He could remind Jeremy about the reason for his admission and try to help him understand this, where possible. Since Jeremy is asking Frank for help to get home, Frank could suggest getting his diabetes stabilised first as an important aspect of his care. Kindness, respect and dignity at all times, while finding opportunities to competently address his immediate caring needs are priorities. Gaining Jeremy's trust and confidence will make this process more manageable. Frank must listen carefully and show an interest in Jeremy's concerns. As an older person who has a dementia diagnosis, Jeremy is suspicious of anything unfamiliar, and his reluctance to get on the bed or to allow anyone to touch him are aspects of this. Sellman (2011) argues that the value of a trusting relationship between nurses and their patients must lie at the heart of effective care delivery. It is important to foster an atmosphere that encourages Jeremy to feel comfortable talking. Frank could suggest that he will speak to the doctor and find out whether an early discharge is possible or check how long it will take to stabilise his diabetes. Providing accurate and relevant information about their reasons for admission and what the likely outcomes may be help patients to make informed decisions. It must not be assumed that because he lives with dementia, Jeremy lacks capacity at all times (Liberati et al., 2023, Lyons, 2023). Frank should talk to Jeremy about his admiral nurse, who is a specialist nurse who cares for patients living with dementia and find out whether a visit may be a useful intervention that could be arranged as soon as possible. It is possible to demonstrate courage and commitment to improve Jeremy's experience while ensuring that he is treated respectfully at all times. Jeremy talks about his wife as if she is still alive. Frank should not take on the task of reminding Jeremy that his wife has passed away; instead the trained admiral nurse will be the best person to deal with this issue (Dening et al., 2022).

Further reading

Felber, S (2023) Triangle of Compassion in Healthcare Communication – From Theory to Evolving Practice: Presenter (s): Steffen Eychmueller, University of Bern, Switzerland. *Patient Education and Counselling*, 109: 147.

Discusses how to apply theoretical approaches to communication practice.

Moorhead, A (2023) Teaching Student Nurses Interprofessional Communication Using Role-Play: An Exploratory Study: Presenter (s): Carmel Quigley, Ulster University, United Kingdom. *Patient Education and Counselling*, 109: 147.

Considers how role play can help learners practise communication skills interprofessionally.

Todt, K (2023) Strategies to Combat Implicit Bias in Nursing. *The American Nurse Journal*, 18 (7): 9–23.

Explores ways that compassion in nursing can be influenced by implicit bias and how to overcome this.

Useful websites

www.zachbeach.com/the-four-components-of-compassion/

Summarises compassion levels under four domains which make them relevant and applicable in any situation.

www.positivepsychology.com/compassion-at-work-leadership/

Gives an overview of compassionate leadership expectations in the workplace.

www.england.nhs.uk/wp-content/uploads/2016/05/cip-yr-3.pdf

Outlines NHS strategy supporting the introduction of the 6Cs.

www.dementiauk.org/for-professionals/how-to-become-an-admiral-nurse/what-do-admiral-nurses-do/

Provides an outline of the work of admiral nurses in their support of patients who live with dementia and their carers, families and other healthcare professionals.

Outlines steps to be followed to ensure that all patients, especially older people are treated with dignity in the NHS.

www.england.nhs.uk/wp-content/uploads/2012/12/compassion-in-practice.pdf

NHS strategic paper that supported the 6Cs implementation in practice.

References

Affengruber, L, Wagner, G, Dobrescu, A, Toromanova, A, Chapman, A, Persad, E, Klerings, I and Gartlehner, G (2023) Values and Preferences of Patients with Depressive Disorders Regarding Pharmacologic and Nonpharmacologic Treatments: A Rapid Review. *Annals of Internal Medicine*, 176 (2): 217–23.

Age UK (2019) Age UK Policy Positions 2019 – A Quick Reference Guide. Available at: www.ageuk.org.uk/globalassets/age-uk/documents/policy-positions/policy_position_quick_reference_guide.pdf (Accessed 17 November 2023).

Akala (2019) *Natives: Race and Class in the Ruins of Empire.* London: Hodder and Stoughton.

Alzheimer's Research UK (2022) What Is Alzheimer's Disease? Available at: www.alzheimersresearchuk.org/wp-content/plugins/mof_bl_0.2.9/downloads/WAD-0522-0524_WEB.pdf (Accessed 17 November 2023).

Alzheimer's Research UK (2023) Types of Dementia. Available at: www.alzheimersresearchuk.org (Accessed 17 November 2023).

Arkan, B, Yılmaz, D and Düzgün, F (2020) Determination of Compassion Levels of Nurses Working at a University Hospital. *Journal of Religion and Health*, 59: 29–39.

Arnett, JJ, Zukauskiene, R, Sugimura, K (2014) The New Life Stage of Emerging Adulthood at Age 18–29 Years, Implications for Mental Health. *The Lancet Psychiatry*, 1 (7): 569–76.

Babaei, S and Taleghani, F (2019) Compassionate Care Challenges and Barriers in Clinical Nurses: A Qualitative Study. *Iranian Journal of Nursing and Midwifery Research*, 24 (3): 213.

Barker, S and Williams, S (2018) Compassionate Communication in Mental Health Care, In Wright, K and McKeown, M (eds) *Essentials of Mental Health Nursing*, Volume 1. London: Sage, pages 297–313.

Başoğul, C and Özgür, G (2016) Role of Emotional Intelligence in Conflict Management Strategies of Nurses. *Asian Nursing Research*, 10 (3): 228–33. doi: 10.1016/j.anr.2016.07.002

Baum, SM, Schader, RM and Owen, SV (2023) *To Be Gifted and Learning Disabled: Strengths Based Strategies for Helping Twice Exceptional Students with LD, ADHD, ASD and More.* London: Routledge.

Beresford, P (2020) 'Mad', Mad Studies and Advancing Inclusive Resistance. *Disability & Society*, 35(8): 1337–42.

Blakley, L, Asher, C, Etherington, A, Maher, J, Wadey, E, Walsh, V and Walker, S (2022) 'Waiting for the Verdict': The Experience of Being Assessed under the Mental Health Act. *Journal of Mental Health*, 31(2): 212–19.

Blodgett, JM, Birch, JM, Musella, M, Harkness, F and Kaushal, A (2022) What Works to Improve Wellbeing? A Rapid Systematic Review of 223 Interventions Evaluated with the Warwick-Edinburgh Mental Well-Being Scales. *International Journal of Environmental Research and Public Health*, 19 (23): 15845.

Borgstrom, E and Pearce, C (2022) End of Life Care and Bereavement. Routledge Resources Online. doi: 10.4324/9780367198459-REPRW14-1

Borschman, R and Marina, J (2019) Sexual Identity and Mental Health in Young People: An Opportunity to Reduce Health Inequality. *The Lancet: Child & Adolescent Health*, 3 (2): 57–9.

Borton, T (1970) *Reach Touch and Teach*. New York: McGraw-Hill.

Bowlby, J (2012) *A Secure Base: Clinical Application of Attachment Theory*. London: Routledge.

Brady, G, Franklin, A, and RIP: STARS Collective (2023) 'I Am More Than Just My Label': Rights, Fights, Validation, and Negotiation. Exploring Theoretical Debates on Childhood Disability with Disabled Young People. *Sociology of Health & Illness*, 45 (6): 1376–92.

Braithwaite, J, Clay-Williams, R, Vecellio, E, Marks, D, Hooper, T, Westbrook, M, Westbrook, J, Blakely, B, Ludlow, K (2016) The Basis of Clinical Tribalism, Hierarchy and Stereotyping: a Laboratory-Controlled Teamwork Experiment. *BMJ Open*, 6 (7): e012467. doi:10.1136/bmjopen-2016-012467

Bramley, L and Matiti, M (2014) How Does It Really Feel to Be in My Shoes? Patients' Experiences of Compassion Within Nursing Care and Their Perceptions of Developing Compassionate Nurses. *Journal of Clinical Nursing*, 23 (19–20): 2790–9.

Breast Cancer Now (2021) Available at: https://breastcancernow.org (Accessed 02 February 2024).

Brett, BM (2023) *The Child–Parent Caregiving Relationship in Later life. Midlife Crisis and the Adult Child*. Bristol: Policy Press, Chapter 1.

Brisenden, S (1986) Independent Living and the Medical Model of Disability. *Disability, Handicap and Society*, 1 (2): 173–8.

Brooks, I (2018) *Organisational Behaviour: Individuals, Groups and Organisation*, fifth edition. Harlow: Pearson.

Brown, M (2022) Accent Discrimination Is Alive and Kicking in England, Study Suggests. *The Guardian*. Available at: www.theguardian.com/uk-news/2022/jun/12/accent-discrimination-is-alive-and-kicking-in-britain-study-suggests (Accessed 16 January 2024).

Brown, R, Martin, D, Hickman, N and Barber, P (2023). *Mental Health Law in England and Wales: A Guide for Mental Health Professionals*. London: Sage.

Brown, TN (2003) Critical Race Theory Speaks to the Sociology of Mental Health: Mental Health Problems Produced by Racial Stratification. *Journal of Health and Social Behavior*, 44 (3): 292–301.

Bunbury, S (2019) Unconscious Bias and the Medical Model: How the Social Model May Hold the Key to Transformative Thinking about Disability Discrimination. *International Journal of Discrimination and the Law*, 19 (1): 26–47.

Burgess, JE, Gorton, KL, Lasiter, S and Patel, SE (2023) The Nurses' Perception of Expressive Touch: An Integrative Review. *Journal of Caring Sciences*, 12 (1): 4.

Burke, JR, Downey, C and Almoudaris, AM (2022) Failure to Rescue Deteriorating Patients: A Systematic Review of Root Causes and Improvement Strategies. *Journal of Patient Safety*, 18 (1): 140–55. doi: 10.1097/PTS.0000000000000720

Carter, L (2019) Communicating Skills in Difficult Situations. In Norman, K *Communication Skills for Nursing and Healthcare Students*. Banbury: Lantern, pages 83–101.

(The) Centre for Ageing Better (2022) The State of Ageing. Available at: ageing-better. org.uk/ (Accessed 17 November 2023).

Challenging Behaviour Foundation (CBF) (2022) Understanding Challenging Behaviour. Available at: www.challengingbehaviour.org.uk/understanding-challenging-behaviour/ (Accessed 17 November 2023).

Chandler, DE and Kram, KE (2005) Applying an Adult Development Perspective to Developmental Networks. *Career Development International*, 10 (6/7): 548–66.

Chapman, K, Dixon, A, Ehrlich, C and Kendall, E (2024) Dignity and the Importance of Acknowledgement of Personhood for People with Disability. *Qualitative Health Research*, 34 (1–2): 141–53.

Cherry, G, Fletcher, I, Shaw, N, O'Sullivan, H (2020) What Impact do Structured Educational Sessions to Increase Emotional Intelligence Have on Medical Students? BEME Guide No. 17. *Medical Teacher*, 34 (1): 11–19.

Chordiya, R, Dolamore, S, Love, JM, Borry, EL, Protonentis, A, Stern, B and Whitebread, G (2023) Staking the Tent at the Margins: Using Disability Justice to Expand the Theory and Praxis of Social Equity in Public Administration. *Administrative Theory & Praxis*: 1–26.

Clarke, D (2022) Death in the UK: Statistics and Facts. Available at: http/www.statista. com/topics/6656/death-in-the-uk/ (Accessed 04 March 2024),

Clemency, C (2021) Disability-Affirmative Integrated Primary Care. *Families, Systems, & Health*, 39 (3): 546.

Clements, C, Farooq, B, Hawton, K, Geulayov, G, Casey, D, Waters, K, Ness, J, Kelly, S, Townsend, E, Appleby, L and Kapur, N (2023) Self-Harm in University Students: A Comparative Analysis of Data from the Multicentre Study of Self-Harm in England. *Journal of Affective Disorders*, 335 (2023): 67–74.

Cooksley, T, Clarke, S, Dean, J, Hawthorn, K, James, A, Tzortzou-Brown, V, Boyle, A (2023) NHS Crisis: Rebuilding the NHS Needs Urgent Action. *British Medical Journal*, 380: 1.

Corr, CA (2018) The Five Stages of Coping with Dying and Bereavement: Strengths, Weaknesses, and Some Alternatives. *Mortality*, 24 (4): 405–17.

Cray, M and Embleton, N (2018) Fathers in the NICU: What Type of Support Do They Need? *Infant*, 14 (4): 129–30.

Crenshaw, K (1989) Demarginalizing the Intersection of Race and Sex: Black Feminist Critique of Antidiscrimination Doctrine, Feminist Theory and Antiracist Politics. *University of Chicago Legal Forum*, pages 139–68.

CYPN (2022) Campaigners Warn of Alarming Rise in Teenage Suicides. Available at: www.cypnow.co.uk/news/article/campaigners-warn-of-alarming-rise-in-teenage-suicides (Accessed 01 February 2024).

D'Antonio, P (2006) History for a Practice Profession. *Nursing Inquiry*, 13 (4): 242–8.

Davidge, G, Brown, L, Lyons, M, Charlotte, B, French, D, van Staa, T and McMillan, B (2023) Principles into Practice: A Qualitative Exploration of the Views and Experiences of Primary Care Staff Regarding Patients Having Access to Their Electronic Health Record. *British Journal of General Practice*, 73 (731): 418–26. doi: 10.399/BJGP.2022.0436

Dening, KH, Aldridge, Z and Hayo, H (2022) Admiral Nursing: Supporting Generalist Nurses to Work with Families Affected by Dementia. *Nursing Standard*, 38 (2): 41–5.

Department of Health and Social Care (2010) Valuing People Now: Summary Report March 2009 – September 2010. Available at: assets.publishing.service.gov.uk/media/5a7cc35340f0b6629523ba98/dh_122387.pdf (Accessed 16 January 2024).

Department of Health and Social Care (2011) Healthy Lives, Healthy People: Update and Way Forward. Available at: www.gov.uk/government/publications/healthy-lives-healthy-people-update-and-way-forward (Accessed 31 January 2024).

Department of Health and Social Care (2022) A Plan for Digital Health and Social Care. Available at: www.gov.uk/government/publications/a-plan-for-digital-health-and-social-care/a-plan-for-digital-health-and-social-care (Accessed 17 November 2023).

Department For Transport (2023) Road Accidents and Safety Statistics. Available at: www.gov.uk/government/collections/road-accidents-and-safety-statistics (Accessed 02 February 2024).

DeRosa, E (2017) Ignorance Is Bliss: Emotion, Politics, and Why Whites Avoid Information About Race. Available at: digitalcommons.lib.uconn.edu/cgi/viewcontent.cgi?article=1545&context=srhonors_theses (Accessed 31 January 2024).

Devlin, S, Healy, O, Leader, G and Hughes, B (2011) Comparison of Behavioral Intervention and Sensory-Integration Therapy in the Treatment of Challenging Behavior. *Journal of Autism and Developmental Disorders*, 41 (10): 1303–20.

De Vries, K (2013) Communicating with Older People with Dementia. *Nursing Older People*, 25 (4): 30–37. doi:10.7748/nop2013.05.25.4.30. e429

Digital Capacity Framework (2015) Building Digital Capability. Available at: www.jisc.ac.uk/building-digital-capability. (Accessed 21 January 2024).

Dolan, P, Kudrna, L and Testoni, S (2017) Definition and Measures of Subjective Wellbeing. Available at: whatworkswellbeing.org/wp-content/uploads/2020/01/SWB-dolan-kudra-Testoni-NOV17-Centre.pdf (Accessed 16 January 2024).

Doran, GT (1981) There's a SMART Way to Write Management's Goals and Objectives. *Management Review*, 70 (11): 35–6.

Doyle, A (2022) What Are Listening Skills? Available at: www.thebalancemoney.com/types-of-listening-skills-with-examples-2063759 (Accessed 16 January 2024).

Drake, R (2018) Dilemmas Of E-Rostering, Old and New: Towards Intelligent Systems? *Nursing Times*, 115 (6): 19–23.

Draper, B and Withall, A (2016) Young Onset Dementia. *Internal Medicine Journal*, 46 (7): 779–86. doi:10.1111/imj.13099

Driscoll J (2007) *Practising Clinical Supervision: A Reflective Approach for Healthcare Professionals*, second edition. Edinburgh: Bailliere Tindall Elsevier.

Dryden, P, Greenshields, S (2020) Communicating with Children and Young People. *British Journal of Nursing*, 29 (2). doi: 10.12968/bjon.2020.29.20.1164

Dunkel, CS, Harbke, C (2017) A Review of Measures of Erikson's Stages of Psychosocial Development: Evidence for a General Factor. *Journal of Adult Development*, 24 (1): 58–76.

Egan, G (1990) *The Skilled Helper: A Systematic Approach to Effective Helping*, fourth edition. California: Thomson Brooks/Cole Publishing.

Ellis-Robinson, T, Slusarz, E, Haji-Georgi, M, Slichko, J, Mohammed, A, Terry, K and Hazell, K (2023) Collaborative Action Research with Diverse Stakeholders: Building the Disability Champions Mentoring Network. *Career Development and Transition for Exceptional Individuals.* Doi: 10.1177/21651434231200176

Fadipe, MF, Aggarwal, S, Johnson, C and Beauchamp, JE (2023) Effectiveness of Online Cognitive Behavioural Therapy on Quality of Life in Adults with Depression: A Systematic Review. *Journal of Psychiatric and Mental Health Nursing*, 30 (5): 885–98.

Farrugia, D (2019) An Exploration of the Perceptions of Mothers and Their Daughters with Intellectual Disability on Forming Relationships, Marriage and Parenting. Master's thesis, University of Malta.

Fisher M and Kieman M (2019) Student Nurses' Lived Experience of Patient Safety and Raising Concerns. *Nurse Education Today*, 77: 1–5.

Fleming, S, Burke, É, Doyle, C, Henderson, K, Horan, P, Byrne, K and Keenan, K (2023) Ensuring Effective Communication When Undertaking a Systematic Health Assessment. *Learning Disability Practice*, 26 (6): e2197

Fletcher, T, Glasper, A, Prudhoe, G, Battrick, C, Coles, L, Weaver, K and Ireland, L (2011) Building the Future: Children's Views on Nurses and Hospital Care. *British Journal of Nursing*, 20 (1): 39–45. doi: 10.12968/ bjon.2011.20.1

Ford, M (2020) New NHSX Chief Nurse Seeks to 'Professionalise' Digital Nursing. *Nursing Times.* Available at: https://www.nursingtimes.net/news/technology/new-nhsx-chief-nurse-seeking-to-professionalise-digital-nursing-13-03-2020/ (Accessed 17 November 2023).

Foseca, LM and Testoni, I (2012) The Emergence of Thanatology and Current Practice in Death Education. *Journal of Death & Dying*, 64 (2): 157–9.

Francis, R (2013) Report of the Mid-Staffordshire NHS Foundation Trust Public Inquiry. Available at: www.gov.uk/government/publications/report-of-the-mid-staffordshire-nhs-foundation-trust-public-inquiry (Accessed 16 January 2024).

Freshwater, D (2007) Teaching and Learning Reflective Practice. In Stickley, T and Basset, T, *Teaching Mental Health*, pages 265–74.

Galanis, E, Hatzigeorgiadis, A, Comoutos, N, Papaioannou, A, Morres, ID and Theodorakis, Y (2022) Effects of a Strategic Self-Talk Intervention on Attention Functions. *International Journal of Sport and Exercise Psychology*, 20 (5): 1368–82.

Gault, I, Shapcott, J, Luthi, A and Reid, G (2016) *Communication in Nursing and Healthcare: A Guide for Compassionate Practice.* London: Sage.

Gibbs, G (2013) Learning by Doing. A Guide to Teaching and Learning Methods. Available at: thoughtsmostlyaboutlearning.files.wordpress.com/2015/12/learning-by-doing-graham-gibbs.pdf (Accessed 18 January 2024).

Giri, A, Aylott, J, Giri, P, Ferguson-Wormley, S and Evans, J (2022) Lived Experience and the Social Model of Disability: Conflicted and Inter-Dependent Ambitions for Employment of People with a Learning Disability and Their Family Carers. *British Journal of Learning Disabilities*, 50 (1): 98–106.

Goldiner, A (2022) Understanding 'Disability' as a Cluster of Disability Models. *The Journal of Philosophy of Disability*, 2 (2022): 28–54.

Goleman, D (2009) *Working with Emotional Intelligence.* London: Bloomsbury.

Gorman, E (2011) Adaptation, Resilience, and Growth After Loss. In Harris, DL (ed) *Counting Our Losses: Reflecting on Change, Loss, and Transition in Everyday Life.* New York: Routledge, pages 225–37.

Gottlieb, L (2012) *Strengths-Based Nursing Care: Health and Healing for Person and Family.* New York: Springer.

Granger, K (2013) Healthcare Staff Must Properly Introduce Themselves to Patients. *BMJ* 2013: 347. doi: 10.1136/bmj.f5833

Harte, V (2022) Development of a Nurse-Led Transport Service for Non-Critical Neonates and Children in Northern Ireland. *Nursing Children and Young People*, 35 (1): 14–19. doi: 10.7748/ncyp.2022.e1426

Hartigan, J (2010) *Race in the 21st Century.* New York: Oxford University Press.

Health Education England (HEE) (2022) Integrated Care. Available at: https://www.hee.nhs.uk/our-work/integrated-care (Accessed 17 November 2023).

Holme, A (2015) Why History Matters to Nursing. *Nurse Education Today*, 35 (5): 635–7.

Holmes, T and Rahe, R (1967) The Social Readjustment Rating Scale. *Journal of Psychosomatic Research*, 11 (2): 213– 18.

Hughes, CA, Morris, JR, Therrien, WJ and Benson, SK (2017) Explicit Instruction: Historical and Contemporary Contexts. *Learning Disabilities Research & Practice*, 32 (3): 40–148.

Hunt, J (2022) *Zero: Eliminating Unnecessary Deaths in a Post-Pandemic NHS.* London: Swift Press.

Hutchings, R (2020) The Impact of Covid-19 on the Use of Digital Technology in the NHS. Nuffield Trust. Available at: www.nuffieldtrust.org.uk/research/the-impact-of-covid-19-on-the-use-of-digital-technology-in-the-nhs (Accessed 13 January 2024).

Isangula, K, Pallangyo, ES, Mbekenga, C, Ndirangu-Mugo, E, Shumba, C (2022). Factors Shaping Good and Poor Nurse–Client Relationships in Maternal and Childcare: A Qualitative Study in Rural Tanzania. *BMC Nursing*, 21 (247). doi: 10.1186/s12912-022-01021-x

Ismael, S, Gibbons, D and Shamini, G (2013) Reducing Inappropriate Accident and Emergency Department Attendances: A Systematic Review of Primary Care Service Interventions. *British Journal of General Practice*, 63 (617): e813–e820.

Jack, K, Levett-Jones, T, Ylonen, A, Ion, R, Pich, J, Fulton, R and Hamshire, C (2021) 'Feel the Fear and Do It Anyway' … Nursing Students Experiences of Confronting Poor Practice. *Nurse Education in Practice*, 56: 1–7. doi: 10.1016/j.nepr.2021.103196.

Jasper, M (2013) *Beginning Reflective Practice*, second edition. Australia: Cengage Learning.

Johns, C (2022) *Becoming a Reflective Practitioner*. London: Wiley-Blackwell.

Jiang, X (2021) 'Introductory Chapter: On the Road Towards the Social-Adaptive Implication of Nonverbal Communication', in Jiang, X (ed) *Types of Nonverbal Communication*, London: IntechOpen. doi:10.5772/intechopen.99869

Kacperck, L (1997) Non-verbal Communication: The Importance of Listening. *British Journal of Nursing*, 6 (5): 275–9.

Karreinen, S, Paananen, H, Kihlström, L, Janhonen, K, Huhtakangas, M, Viita-aho, M and Tynkkynen, L-K (2023) Living Through Uncertainty: A Qualitative Study of Leadership and Resilience in Primary Health Care during COVID-19. *BMC Health Services Research*, 23 (233): 1–13.

Kegan, R (1994) *In Over Our Heads: The Mental Demands of Modern Life*. Massachusetts: Harvard University Press.

Kerr, D, Martin, P, Furber, L, Winterburn, S, Milnes, S, Nielsen, A and Strachan, P (2022) Communication Skills Training for Nurses: Is it Time For a Standardised Nursing Model? *Patient Education and Counselling*, 105 (7): 1970–5.

King, LM, Lacey, A, Hunt, J (2022) Applying Communication Skills in the Provision of Family-Centred Care: A Reflective Account. *Nursing Children and Young People*, 34 (2): 22–7. doi: 10.7748/ncyp.2021.e1388

King's Fund (2022) An Introduction to Leading with Kindness and Compassion in Health and Social Care. Available at: www.kingsfund.org.uk/courses/introduction-kindness-compassion-health-and-social-care (Accessed 17 November 2023).

Kleemola, E, Leino-Kilpi, H and Numminen, O (2020) Care Situations Demanding Moral Courage: Content Analysis of Nurses' Experiences. *Nursing Ethics*, 27 (3): 714–25.

Kolb, DA (1984) *Experiential Learning: Experience as the Source of Learning and Development*. New Jersey, Prentice-Hall.

Kubler-Ross, E (1969) *On Death and Dying. What the Dying Have to Say to Teach Doctors, Nurses, Clergy and Their Own Families*. New York: Scribner.

Lawson, A and Beckett, AE (2021) The Social and Human Rights Models of Disability: Towards a Complementarity Thesis. *The International Journal of Human Rights*, 25 (2): 348–79.

Ledger, S, McCormack, N, Walmsley, J, Tilley, E and Davies, I (2022) 'Everyone Has a Story to Tell': A Review of Life Stories in Learning Disability Research and Practice. *British Journal of Learning Disabilities*, 50 (4): 484–93.

Legislation.gov.uk (2005a) Disability and Discrimination Act (DDA). Available at: www.legislation.gov.uk/ukpga/2005/13/notes/division/2#:~:text=The%20DDA%2C%20as%20originally%20enacted,disposal%20and%20management%20of%20premises (Accessed 01 February 2024).

Legislation.gov.uk (2005b) Mental Capacity Act. Available at: www.gov.uk/government/publications/mental-capacity-act-code-of-practice (Accessed 04 March 2024).

Legislation.gov.uk (2010) Equality Act 2010 c. 15. Available at www.legislation.gov.uk/ukpga/2010/15/contents (Accessed 17 November 2023).

Legislation.gov.uk (2012) Health and Social Care Act Available at: https://www.legislation.gov.uk/ukpga/2012/7/contents (Accessed 31 January 2024).

Legislation.gov.uk (2014a) Care Act 2014 c. 23. Available at: www.legislation.gov.uk/ukpga/2014/23/contents/ (Accessed 17 November 2023).

Legislation.gov.uk (2014b) Social Services and Wellbeing (Wales) Act. Available at: www.legislation.gov.uk/anaw/2014/4/contents (Accessed 17 November 2023).

Legislation.gov.uk (2022) Health and Social Care Act c. 31. Available at: www.legislation.gov.uk/ukpga/2022/31/contents/enacted(Accessed 01 February 2024).

Levenson, MR and Crumpler, CA (1996) Three Models of Adult Development. *Human Development*, 39 (3): 135–49.

Lewis, P, Gaffney, RJ and Wilson, NJ (2017) A Narrative Review of Acute Care Nurses' Experiences Nursing Patients with Intellectual Disability: Underprepared, Communication Barriers and Ambiguity about the Role of Caregivers. *Journal of Clinical Nursing*, 26 (11–12): 1473–84.

Liberati, E, Richards, N, Ratnayake, S, Gibson, J and Martin, G (2023) Tackling the Erosion of Compassion in Acute Mental Health Services. *BMJ*, (2023): 382. doi: 10.1136/bmj-2022-073055

Lim, M, Eres, R, Peck, C (2019) The Young Australian Loneliness Survey: Understanding Loneliness in Adolescence and Young Adulthood. The Iverson Health Innovation and Research Institute. Swinbourne University of Technology. Available at: www.vichealth.vic.gov.au/sites/default/files/The-young-Australian-loneliness-survey-Report.pdf (Accessed 17 January 2024).

Littler, N (2019) A Qualitative Study Exploring School Nurses' Experiences of Safeguarding Adolescents. *British Journal of School Nursing*. 14 (4):169–76.

Luft, J and Ingham, H (1955) The Johari Window as a Graphic Model of Interpersonal Awareness. *Proceedings of the Western Training Laboratory in Group Development*. Los Angeles: UCLA.

Lyons, K (2023) Could You Be a Consultant Admiral Nurse for Frailty? Kerry Lyons Talks about Her New Post in Dementia UK's First Frailty-Specific Nursing Service and Her Career So Far. *Nursing Older People*, 35 (4): 18–19.

Marmara, J, Zarate, D, Vassallo, J, Patten, R and Stavropoulos, V (2022) Warwick Edinburgh Mental Well-Being Scale (WEMWBS): Measurement Invariance across Genders and Item Response Theory Examination. *BMC Psychology*, 10 (1): 1–17.

Maslow, A (1970) *Motivation and Personality*, second edition. New York: Harper and Row.

MBRRACE-UK (2020) Saving Lives, Improving Mothers' Care. Available at: www.npeu.ox.ac.uk/assets/downloads/mbrrace-uk/reports/maternal-report-2022/MBRRACE-UK_Maternal_CORE_Report_2022_v10.pdf (Accessed 31 January 2024).

Mendes, AMFADS, Brás, SCN, Marques, RMD and Pontífice-Sousa, P (2022) Therapeutic Touch in Nursing Care: A Conceptual Analysis. *Acta Paulista de Enfermagem*, 35: eAPE00706.

MENCAP (nd) Learning Disability Explained. Available at: www.mencap.org.uk/learning-disability-explained (Accessed 01 February 2024).

Merz, S, Jaehn, P, Mena, E, Pöge, K, Strasser, S, Saß, AC, Rommel, A, Bolte, G and Holmberg, C (2023) Intersectionality and Eco-social Theory: A Review of Potentials for Public Health Knowledge and Social Justice. *Critical Public Health*, 33 (2): 125–34.

Misselbrook, D (2014) W Is for Wellbeing and the WHO Definition of Health. *British Journal of General Practice*, 64 (628): 582.

Morgan, S, Gibson, F, Aldiss, S and Porter, L (2022) Effective Transition of Young People with Long-Term Conditions into Adult Services. *Nursing Children and Young People*, 35 (1): 34–42. doi: 10.7748/ncyp. 2022.e1439

Mueller, Jennifer C (2020) Racial Ideology or Racial Ignorance? An Alternative Theory of Racial Cognition. *Sociological Theory*, 38 (2): 142–69.

Neuwirth, LS, Jobvic, S, Mukherji, BR (2021) Re-Imagining Higher Education (HE) During and Post Covid-19: Challenges and Opportunities. *Journal of Adult and Continuing Education* 27 (2): 141–56.

NHS (2023) Communicating with Someone with Dementia. Available at: www.nhs.uk/conditions/dementia/living-with-dementia/communication (Accessed 17 November 2023).

NHS England (2012) The 6Cs of Nursing. Available at: www.england.nhs.uk/6cs/wp-content/uploads/sites/25/2015/03/introducing-the-6cs.pdf (Accessed 17 November 2023).

NHS England (2023) Delivery Plan for Recovering Access to Primary Care. Available at: www.england.nhs.uk/publication/delivery-plan-for-recovering-access-to-primary-care/ (Accessed 22 January 2024).

NHS England (2024) e-Learning for Healthcare. Available at: https://portal.e-lfh.org.uk/ (Accessed 04 March 2024).

NHS England and NHS Improvement (2019) Information Sharing Policy. Available at: https://www.england.nhs.uk/wp-content/uploads/2019/10/information-sharing-policy-v4.1.pdf (Accessed 03 February 2024).

NHS England and NHS Improvement (2020) Integrating care: Next Steps to Building Strong and Effective Integrated Care Systems across England. Available at: www.england.nhs.uk/publication/integrating-care-next-steps-to-building-strong-and-effective-integrated-care-systems-across-england/ (Accessed 31 January 2024).

NHS England and NHS Improvement (2021a) Equity and Equality: Guidance for Local Maternity Systems. Available at: www.england.nhs.uk/publication/equity-and-equality-guidance-for-local-maternity-systems/ (Accessed 04 March 2024).

NHS England and NHS Improvement (2021b) Online Library of Quality, Service Improvement and Redesign Tools: SBAR Communication Tool. Available at: www.england.nhs.uk/improvement-hub/wp-content/uploads/sites/44/2017/11/SBAR-Implementation-and-Training-Guide.pdf (Accessed 04 March 2024).

NICE (National Institute for Health and Care Excellence) (2015) Challenging Behaviour and Learning Disabilities: Prevention and Interventions for People with Learning

Disabilities Whose Behaviour Challenges (NICE Guideline NG11) Available at: https:// www.nice.org.uk/guidance/ng11 (Accessed 01 February 2024).

NICE (National Institute for Health and Care Excellence) (2019) End of Life Care for Adults: Service Delivery. London: NICE.

NICE (National Institute for Health and Care Excellence) (2021) Dementia. Available at: cks.nice.org.uk/topics/dementia (Accessed 17 November 2023).

Nicholson, C (2016) How Do We Facilitate Carers' Involvement in Decision-Making? *Nursing Older People*, 28 (3): 14–14. doi: 10.7748/nop.28.3.14.s21

NMC (2018) The Code: Professional Standards of Practice and Behaviour for Nurses, Midwives and Nursing Associates. Available at: www.nmc.org.uk/globalassets/ sitedocuments/nmc-publications/nmc-code.pdf (Accessed 17 November 2023).

NMC (2022) Raising Concerns and Whistleblowing. Available at: www.nmc.org.uk/standards/ guidance/raising-concerns-guidance-for-nurses-and-midwives (Accessed 17 November 2023).

NMC (2023) Realising Professionalism: Standards for Education and Training Part 3: Standards for Pre-Registration Midwifery Programmes. Available at: https://heiw. nhs.wales/files/once-for-wales/once-for-wales-2020-midwifery-documents/overall-introduction-and-overview-of-all-wales-elements/ (Accessed 04 March 2024).

Noone, PA (2017) The Holmes-Rahe Stress Inventory. *Occupational Medicine*, 67 (97): 581–2.

Nordquist, P (2021) Social Scripts. Relationality and Donor Conception. *Sociology*, 55 (4): 677–95.

Norman, K (2015) How Mentors Can Influence the Values, Behaviours, and Attitudes of Nursing Staff through Positive Professional Socialisation. *Nursing Management*, 22 (8): 33–9.

Norman, K (2019) *Communication Skills for Nursing and Healthcare Students*. Banbury: Lantern.

Nguyen, LH, Dawson, JE, Brooks, M, Khan, JS and Telusca, N (2023) Disparities in Pain Management. *Anesthesiology Clinics*, 41 (2): 471–88.

O'Luanaigh, P (2015) Becoming a Professional: What Is the Influence of Registered Nurses on Nursing Students' Learning in the Clinical Environment. *Nurse Education in Practice*, 15 (6): 450-6.

O'Malley, E-J, Hansjee S, Abdel-Hadi, B, Kendrick, E and Lok, S (2022) A Covid-19 Virtual Ward Model: A Preliminary Retrospective Clinical Evaluation from a UK District General Hospital. *Journal of Primary Care & Community Health*, 13: 1–7. doi: 10.1177/21501319211066667

ONS (Office for National Statistics) (2021a) Birth Characteristics in England and Wales. Available at: www.ons.gov.uk/peoplepopulationandcommunity/birthsdeathsandmarriages/ livebirths/datasets/birthcharacteristicsinenglandandwales (Accessed 31 January 2024).

ONS (2021b) Mental Health of Children, Adolescents and Adults: Available at: https:// www.ons.gov.uk/peoplepopulationandcommunity/healthandsocialcare/mentalhealth (Accessed 31 January 2024).

ONS (Office for National Statistics) (2021c) Profile of the Older Population Living in England and Wales in 2021 and Changes since 2011. Available at: www.ons.gov.uk/

peoplepopulationandcommunity/birthsdeathsandmarriages/ageing/articles/profileof theolderpopulationlivinginenglandandwalesin2021andchangessince2011/2023-04-03 (Accessed 31 January 2024).

ONS (Office for National Statistics) (2022a) Monthly Mortality Analysis, England and Wales. Available at: https://www.ons.gov.uk/peoplepopulationandcommunity/ birthsdeathsandmarriages/deaths/bulletins/monthlymortalityanalysisenglandandwales/ previousReleases (Accessed 04 March 2024).

ONS (Office for National Statistics) (2022b) UK National Wellbeing Scales. Available at: www. ons.gov.uk/peoplepopulationandcommunity/wellbeing (Accessed 17 November 2023).

Öztürk, A and Kaçan, H (2022) Compassionate Communication Levels of Nursing Students: Predictive Role of Empathic Skills and Nursing Communication Course. *Perspectives in Psychiatric Care*, 58 (1): 248–55.

Papadopoulos, R (2011) Transcultural Nursing: The Vehicle for the Delivery of Much Needed Compassionate and Culturally Competent Care for All. International Conference on Transcultural Nursing. Available at: repository.mdx.ac.uk/item/8412w (Accessed 31 January 2024).

Pajakoski, E, Rannikko, S, Leino-Kilpi, H and Numminen, O (2021) Moral Courage in Nursing – An Integrative Literature Review. *Nursing and Health Sciences*, 23 (3): 570–85.

Panorama team and Joseph Lee (2022) 'Toxic Culture' of Abuse at Mental Health Hospital Revealed by BBC Secret Filming, BBC News. Available at: www.bbc.co.uk/news/ uk-63045298 (Accessed 17 November 2023).

Parkes, CM (1972) *Stages of Bereavement. Bereavement: Studies in Grief in Adult Life.* London Tavistock Clinic Series.

Patel, A, Piggot, K, Wong, A, Patel, A, Patel, M, Liu, Y, Dhesy-Thind, S, Wasi, P and You, JJ (2018) Role of Allied Health Care Professionals in Goals of Care Discussions with Hospitalised Patients and Perceived Barriers. A Cross Sectional Survey. *Canadian Medical Association Open Access Journal*, 6 (2): 241–7.

Pérez-Duarte Mendiola, P (2022) How to Communicate with Children, According to Health Play Specialists in the United Kingdom: A Qualitative Study. *Journal of Child Health Care.* doi: 10.117713674935221109113

Protection of Vulnerable Groups Scotland (2007) Available at: www.gov.scot/ binaries/content/documents/govscot/publications/consultation-analysis/2016/07/ protection-vulnerable-groups-scotland-act-2007-section-35-2-3/documents/00503540- pdf/00503540-pdf/govscot%3Adocument/00503540.pdf (Accessed 01 February 2024).

Purtle, J, Nelson, KL, Counts, NZ and Yudell, M (2020) Population-Based Approaches to Mental Health: History, Strategies, and Evidence. *Annual Review of Public Health*, 41 (April): 201–21.

Rabbit, A and Coyne, I (2012) Childhood Obesity: Nurses' Role in Addressing the Epidemic. *British Journal of Nursing*, 21 (12): 731–5. doi: 10.12968/bjon.2012.21.12.731

Raleigh, V and Holmes, J (2021) The Health of People from Ethnic Minority Groups in England. Kings Fund. Available at: www.kingsfund.org.uk/publications/health-people- ethnic-minority-groups-england (Accessed 17 January 2024).

RCN (Royal College of Nursing) (2015) The 6Cs of Nursing. Available at: /rcni.com/nursing-standard/revalidation/6cs-of-nursing-32156 (Accessed 17 November 2023).

RCN (Royal College of Nursing) (2022a) Staffing Crisis in the NHS. Available at: www.rcn.org.uk/news-and-events/news/uk-staffing-crisis-jeopardising-safe-care-nhs-survey-300322 (Accessed 22 January 2024).

RCN (Royal College of Nursing) (2022b) Top Tips for Video Consultations. Available at: www.rcn.org.uk/magazines/Advice/2022/May/Top-tips-for-digital-consultations (Accessed 17 November 2023).

Robichaux, C, Tietze, M, Stokes, F and McBride, S (2019) Reconceptualising the Electronic Health Record for a New Decade: A Caring Technology? *Advances in Nursing Science*, 42 (3): 193–205.

Rogers, C (1957) *Client-Centred Therapy: Its Current Practice, Implications and Theory.* London: Constable.

RQIA (The Regulation and Quality Improvement Authority) (2016) Adult Safeguarding Operational Procedures. Available at: www.rqia.org.uk/RQIA/files/b1/b197727b-f21c-4e93-a60f-1775bb2e3c4a.pdf (Accessed 17 November 2023).

Schon, DA (1991) *The Reflective Practitioner: How Professionals Think in Action.* Aldershot: Ashgate Publishing.

Schut, MSH (1999) The Dual Process Model of Coping with Bereavement: Rationale and Description. *Death Studies*, 23 (3): 197-224.

SCIE (2011) What Is Personalisation? Available at: www.scie.org.uk/personalisation/introduction/what-is (Accessed 17 November 2023).

SCIE (2022a) Integrated Care. Available at: www.scie.org.uk/integrated-care/definition-legislation (Accessed 17 November 2023).

SCIE (2022b) Prevention and Healthcare. Available at: www.scie.org.uk/integrated-care/research-practice/activities/prevention-self-care/#:~:text=Prevention%20helps%20individuals% (Accessed 04 March 2024).

SCIE (2022b) Strengths-Based Social Care. Available at: www.scie.org.uk/strengths-based-approaches/young-people/ (Accessed 01 February 2024).

Segal, J (1997) *Raising Your Emotional Intelligence. A Practical Guide.* New York: Holt.

Sellman, D (2011) *What Makes a Good Nurse – Why the Virtues Are Important for Nursing.* London: Jessica Kingsley Publishers.

Sharma, D, Levron, E, Yang Ye (2022) 50 Years of British Accent Bias: Stability and Lifespan Change in Attitudes to Accents. *English World-Wide*, 43 (2): 135–166.

Sharma, N and Gupta, V (2022) *Therapeutic Communication.* Florida: StatPearls Publishing.

Shields, L (2015) 'What Is Family-Centred Care?' *European Journal of Person-Centred Healthcare*, 13 (2): 139–44.

Sickle Cell Society (2021) No One's listening – A Report. Available at: www.sicklecellsociety.org/no-ones-listening/ (Accessed 17 November 2023).

Simons, G and Baldwin, DS (2021) A Critical Review of the Definition of 'Wellbeing' for Doctors and Their Patients in a Post Covid-19 Era. *International Journal of Social Psychiatry*, 67 (8): 984–91.

Smith, M (2008) Racism and Motivational Ignorance. *The ARDEN Review*, 1 (1): 3–14.

Stenholm, S, Westerlund, H, Head, J, Hyde, M, Kawachi, I, Pentti, J, Kivimäki, M, Vahtera, J (2014) Comorbidity and Functional Trajectories from Midlife to Old Age: The Health and Retirement Study. *The Journals of Gerontology: Series A*, 70 (3): 332–8. doi: 10.1093/gerona/glu113

Stockwell, F (1972) *The Unpopular Patient*. Beckenham: Croom Helm.

Su, JJ, Masika, GM, Paguio, JT and Redding, SR (2020) Defining Compassionate Nursing Care. *Nursing Ethics*, 27 (2): 480–93.

Thompson, N (2021) *Anti-Discriminatory Practice: Equality, Diversity and Social Justice*, seventh edition. London: Bloomsbury/BASW.

Thompson, S and Thompson, N (2023) *The Critically Reflective Practitioner*. London: Bloomsbury.

Todt, K (2023) Strategies to Combat Implicit Bias in Nursing. *The American Nurse Journal*, 18 (7): 9–23.

Topel, E (2019) Preparing the Healthcare Workforce to Deliver the Digital Future: An Independent Report on Behalf of the Secretary of State for Health and Social Care. NHS. Available at: topol.hee.nhs.uk/wp-content/uploads/HEE-Topol-Review-2019.pdf (Accessed 18 January 2024).

Underman Boggs, K (2022) *Interpersonal Relationships: Professional Communication Skills for Nurses*, ninth edition. Missouri: Elsevier.

Watson, NA (2019) Communication and Diversity. In Norman, K *Communication Skills for Nurses and Healthcare Students*. Banbury: Lantern, pages 105–24.

Watson, NA (2001) Equal Value, Equal Care: Differences and Diversity, Primary Care Perspectives, in Watson, NA and Wilkinson, C *Nursing in Primary Care: A Handbook for Students*. Basingstoke: Palgrave, pages 119–37.

West, P, Van Riper, M, Wyatt, G, Lehto, R, Douglas, SN, Robbins, L (2020) Adaptation to Technology Use in Families of Children with Complex Communication Needs: An Integrative Review and Family Theory Application. *Journal of Family Nursing*, 26 (2): 153–78. doi: 10.1177/107484072091553

Wilkinson, C and Maurimootoo, S (2001) Promoting Mental Health in Primary Care, in Watson, NA and Wilkinson, C (2001) *Nursing in Primary Care: A Handbook for Students*. Basingstoke: Palgrave, pages 237–62.

Williams, M (2023) Addressing Challenges in End-of-Life Communication with Patients and Families. *Nursing Standard*, 38 (6): 78–82.

Wood, D, Crapnell, T, Lau, L, Bennet, A, Lotstein, D, Ferris, M and Kuo, A (2018) Emerging Adulthood as a Critical Stage in the Life Course, in Halfon, N, Forrest, C, Lerner, R, Faustman, E (eds) *Handbook of Life Course Health Development*. Cham: Springer, pages 123–43.

WHO (World Health Organization) (2020a) Cancer Incidence, Global Perspectives. Geneva: WHO.

World Health Organization (WHO) (2020b) Coronavirus Disease (COVID-19) Pandemic. Available at: www.who.int/europe/emergencies/situations/covid-19 (Accessed 26 January 2024).

WHO (World Health Organization) (2020c) Primary Care. Geneva: WHO.

WHO (World Health Organization) (2021a) Global Status Report on the Public Health Response to Dementia: Available at: iris.who.int/bitstream/handle/10665/344701/9789240033245-eng.pdf (Accessed 24 January 2024).

WHO (World Health Organization) (2021b) Mental Health. Geneva: WHO.

WHO (World Health Organization) (2022) Palliative Care. Geneva: WHO.

World Cancer Research Fund (WCRF) 2020) Preventing Cancer, Saving Lives. Available at www.wcrf-uk.org (Accessed 26 January 2024).

Index

Note: Page numbers in *italics* and **bold** representing figures and tables respectively.